the CanCell
Controversy

PEOPLE
AGAINST
CANCER

P.O. Box 10 • Otho, IA 50569-0010

Phone 515-972-4444 • Fax 515-972-4415

the CanCell Controversy

WHY IS A POSSIBLE CURE FOR CANCER BEING SUPPRESSED?

Louise B. Trull

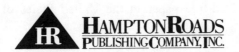

HAMPTON ROADS
PUBLISHING COMPANY, INC.

Hampton Roads Publishing Company, Inc.
891 Norfolk Square
Norfolk, VA 23502
Or call: (804) 459-2453
FAX: (804) 455-8907

If you are unable to order this book from your local bookseller, you may order directly from the publisher.
Call 1-800-766-8009, toll-free.

Cover design by Patrick Smith

ISBN 1-878901-76-1

10 9 8 7 6 5 4 3 2 1

Printed on acid-free paper in the United States of America

To my Mother

Augustina Boehs Biedenbach

The credulous believe too much,
the scientific too little.

Albert Abrams, M.D.
(1863-1924)

Preface

There is a universal law of repair that belongs right alongside the one that says, "If it ain't broke, don't fix it," and it says, "If you don't know what's wrong, you can't fix it." After almost ten years of looking at the cancer industry, I have concluded that our so-called cancer experts don't know what cancer really is and cannot possibly find a sure cure for it until they do.

I consider myself one of the lucky cancer victims. Almost ten years ago, during a routine physical checkup, a radiologist identified what he considered a cancer on a mammogram and that resulted in my having a modified mastectomy. Because the cancer was thought to be in its very early stages and there were no signs of its having spread to the lymph system, no radiation or chemotherapy was recommended. That's why I consider myself to be a lucky cancer victim. Back then, when all I knew about cancer was what I read and believed in literature based upon opinion expressed by the American Cancer Society, I'm sure I would have complacently followed any recommendations my attending physicians would have given. If they had told me to have chemotherapy "just to be sure and as a preventive measure," as many women have been told, I believe I would have done that and I would not be alive today, just as many who followed such doctors' orders are no longer living.

I am what friends consider a health nut. After spending three years as a high school English teacher, I married and became a stay-at-home wife and mother. I took my homemaking job as seriously as I had taken my teaching job. Since I considered myself to be in charge of the family health, I read a lot about nutrition, exercise, and keeping healthy, and I gradually put what I learned into practice. I think education and experience combined to pay dividends for my family in the form of good health.

So what caused the cancer? My friends were astonished. They considered me the last person they knew who would be a candidate for cancer. Because I am a very private person, few were aware of the constant personal stress that dominated my life and which I now believe initiated it.

But what is the process of cancer? How does it grow from stress to become a killing agent? How and when does the transformation from a healthy cell to a cancer cell take place? These questions plagued me. I had a basic need to understand the how and why of this thing called cancer that dared to invade and threaten me for the rest of my life. I felt I needed to know what cancer really is before I could track its cause, and that's when my understanding of the true nature of the forces that dominate life began.

I had absolutely no background in scientific misinformation to hamper me. I did have a wonderful Latin Grammar School education that teamed with a genetic gift for analytical reasoning and deduction that enabled me to search and find answers to the questions I couldn't ignore.

A couple of health-nut friends of mine, an old college friend and her husband, heard about CanCell and told me about it. I think they were concerned about me and perhaps thought my days were numbered due to my bout with cancer. They had heard a tape by Ed Sopcak (pronounced *Soap-chak*), thought it made a lot of sense and passed it on to me. I contacted Sopcak and we had several long phone conversations during which he explained his hypothesis of cancer. This dedicated man, free of charge, spent more time and effort educating me about cancer than any physician to whom I had paid thousands of dollars ever did. He told me about energy and vibrational frequencies and their damaging effect on cells. It sounded like voodoo medicine to me, but I listened. I thought I had never heard about all of this before. Then I began to remember my grade school teachers trying to explain energy and the constant movement of all atoms in all matter. I never fully comprehended that theory when I was a child and finally accepted it on blind faith, never expecting it to become a practical part of my life.

Then two more friends, who have been studying alternative medical practices for years, assured me that some very well-respected scientists, physicians, and dentists had discovered the forces of energy and vibrational frequencies on cells long ago. They gave me the basic educational foundation I needed to begin to understand cancer by lending me their precious books and patiently explaining the difficult-to-comprehend subject of energy.

In the early 1930s, around the time that a student named Jim Sheridan became fascinated by his own chemical experiments, the scientific world was awakening in full force to this controlling phenomenon, energy and electrons. Several Nobel Prizes had been awarded for discoveries in the field. When practical applications of the findings were attempted by physicians and dentists, however, the established medical industry apparently would not accept the hypothesis they could not understand and displayed contempt for any efforts by practitioners to use the new information. That ultimately intimidated the medical community into virtually abandoning it in general practice.

Ed Sopcak, inspired by the work of Jim Sheridan and the results of Entelev and aware of the Electron Theory, put the knowledge to work and came up with CanCell. He met with the same opposition that stifled medical practitioners over sixty years ago, Nobel Prizes be damned. It seems obvious that both Entelev and CanCell have cured cancers, but, because the cancer industry cannot explain why, it refuses to accept the fact of the cures.

Then I read about physicist Richard Feynman, who died in 1990 at seventy-two and whose life is described in James Glick's book *Genius: The Life and Science of Richard Feynman*. In the book section of *Time* magazine's December 7, 1992, issue, in an article entitled "The Physicist As Magician," Michael D. Lemonick wrote:

. . .He was a physicist's physicist who saw more

deeply into the workings of nature than anyone but Einstein and perhaps a handful of others. His greatest achievement was the theory of quantum electrodynamics, which described the behavior of subatomic particles, atoms, light, electricity and magnetism. . .

. . .He was more interested in getting the solution than in doing the problem according to the rules, and he often ended up reinventing physics as he went. . .Instead of using conventional calculations, he invented "Feynman diagrams," arrows and squiggles that mapped the comings and goings of particles so effectively that they are now a standard tool of physics.

People are dying of cancer every day. Our first priority should be to stop the dying with whatever tools are at hand. If we don't understand why those tools work, let us first use them, stop the dying, and then figure out why they work. The results are more important than understanding the why. If patients choose to look at CanCell results and take a chance on that treatment, it should be their privilege to do so. If they look at the results of traditional treatment and choose to take a chance on that, it should be their privilege to do so. It is as simple as that. Then the ACS, the NCI and the FDA can compile statistics on the results and proceed to untangle the *why* of those results in their own good time.

Contents

Documents

1. **Cancer: A Protein Disease** by Phillip W. Maly, O.D. From information obtained from J. Sheridan, May 4, 1990. Chapter 2.

2. **CanCell/Entelev** by the American Cancer Society Cancer Response System. Printed on 12/16/91, re-typed copy. Chapter 3.

3. **Letter** dated October 2, 1990, from Ven L. Narayanan, Ph.D., Chief, Drug Synthesis & Chemistry Branch, National Cancer Institute, to James V. Sheridan. Chapter 3.

4. **Letter** dated October 15, 1990, from James V. Sheridan to Dr. Narayanan. Chapter 3.

5. **Letter** dated December 21, 1990, and NCI Developmental Therapeutics Program test results from Michael R. Boyd, M.D., Ph.D., to James V. Sheridan. Chapter 3.

6. **The History of Entelev/CanCell** by James V. Sheridan, June 1990, re-typed copy. Chapter 4.

7. **Letter** dated January 7, 1963, from R.S. Davidson, Chief, Biosciences Research of Battelle Columbus Laboratories to W.A. Allen, Secretary, Else U. Pardee Foundation, re-typed copy certified by Mr. Davidson, July 28, 1990. Chapter 4.

8. **Note of termination** of association of Entelev and CanCell, written by Edward J. Sopcak, June 15, 1992. Chapter 5.

9. **The Technology of Entelev, IND-20258 and CanCell, an Identical Material, patent pending**, by J. Sheridan, Third Printing, November 1991. Chapter 5.

10. **Important Information About CanCell**, insert in all supplies of the material, re-typed copy. Chapter 6.

11. **Dietary Recommendations**, re-typed. Chapter 6.

12. **CanCell Reorder Form**. Chapter 6.

13. **Judgment and Order** of Civil Contempt and for Enforcement of Permanent Injunction Against Edward J. Sopcak. Epilogue.

Introduction

Over sixty years have passed since James V. Sheridan first observed a chemical reaction called rhythmic banding in an analytical chemistry laboratory at Carnegie Tech that launched his life-long search for a cancer cure. Fascinated by the Debye Theory, published in 1927, he researched its validity by determining the effect of changes in dielectric constant on reactions between positive and negative ions. Combining the first event with the new technology, he theorized the possibility of a chemical control that might alter the pathway of energy flow and production in the respiratory system to cause or cure a cancer. Years of research culminated in the birth of the Entelev project on September 6, 1936.

Does this obscure Michigan chemist's formula, Entelev, hold the answer to alleviating this scourge of mankind? Or is it just the first giant step to the ultimate answer? Has Edward J. Sopcak, Michigan metallurgist who was inspired by Sheridan's work but who believes the basic cause of cancer to be cell-damaging vibrational frequencies, carried Sheridan's hypothesis to its ultimate conclusion and made CanCell the cure of choice?

Are all of our modern cancer experts wrong in their conception of the basic nature of the disease?

Are the three organizations that directly or indirectly control investigation, research, testing, and approval of new cancer cures preventing an honest scientific examination of each man's basic hypothesis? Has fund-raising and appropriation fixing become a growth industry that finally superseded the cancer research for which they were created? Are drug companies, hospitals, doctors, so-called health insurance companies, and other members of the giant medical service industry purposefully engaged in protecting their economic investments in conventional treatments at the expense of finding a sure cure for cancer; or are they unwittingly caught up in a system hopelessly mired in its own outdated protocol that stifles all research that is not based on accepted conventional theories, right or wrong?

Is Ed Sopcak, who manufactured and distributed CanCell free of charge to cancer patients who requested it, guilty of performing a criminal act of defiance; or is he an unsung hero?

Is CanCell on a mission of mercy or a gigantic hoax? Does it work? Does CanCell deserve a realistic clinical evaluation? It is a time for judgment.

1
The Medical Service Industry

Health care and medical service. Drug companies,
so-called health insurance, medical schools, doctors,
and hospitals. The Electron Theory.

In attempting to explore CanCell as a cancer cure, we
need to understand how today's medical service industry
operates. This knowledge is vital to understanding why
CanCell has never been given a valid clinical testing by
the established hierarchy of U.S. medicine. Indeed, most
people have never heard of it. Some cancer patients who
have the wisdom to look around and see that conventional
treatment is not working and have the courage to trust their
own instincts and the financial ability to do so seek
alternative treatment outside the country. Some others, who
used CanCell, vow it saved their lives.

The treatment both James Sheridan, the creator of Entelev,
and Edward Sopcak, the developer of CanCell, report to
have received at the hands of medical research organizations
and regulatory agencies must be termed bizarre. They claim
their treatment was inspired, controlled, and orchestrated by
the medical service industry. If true, their stories of mis-
conduct on the part of the medical leadership of our country
compares to the most blatant political intrigues and cover-up
scandals of the nation's history.

They paint a picture of conspiracy that may have deprived
cancer victims of the treatment that could have saved their
lives. They present a scenario that is alleged to have been
inspired by the medical community's promotion of their

own established medical treatments as the only acceptable treatments of cancer, initiated by the drug companies, sold to the medical schools, perpetuated by the so-called health insurance companies, and endured by cancer patients in docile compliance with doctors' orders. People tolerate the system because they are afraid to trust their own observations of failed medical practice, and treatment accepted by the system is the only treatment their medical insurance will cover.

It is a gross misnomer to use the term "health care industry" when referring to that area of business which includes all medical personnel from physicians and dentists to auxiliary workers, drug manufacturers and suppliers, hospitals, and health insurance companies. The companies and people involved in that industry provide medical services, and it should be called what it truly is, the "medical service industry."

Health care can be provided to individuals only by themselves, completely apart from the medical services and products bought from the professionals, their suppliers, and support systems. Health care is not provided by health insurance companies; they provide only for medical services. Such insurance should be called what it really is: "medical service insurance."

Most health care is provided by diet and is bought at the grocery store and the health food store; the rest must be provided by individuals for themselves in the form of exercise, adequate rest, and sensible life styles, and it is free. Also included in health care is a commitment to keep current about health and medical information so that an intelligent judgment can be made in case medical service is needed.

Medical service is expensive. Health care is inexpensive. Buying good nutritious food to maintain good health is the cheapest way to feed ourselves. Walking or riding a bicycle instead of using transportation is the best and cheapest kind of exercise needed to keep physically and mentally fit. Diet, exercise, sanitary living conditions, and isolation from communicable diseases are the foundations of health care, and these cannot be provided by insurance or become the responsibility of anyone but ourselves. This lesson must begin in our homes and be nurtured in our schools if we are to become a nation of healthy individuals.

The medical service industry should be ready in a stand-by capacity to take care of accidents and disease, which will dramatically decrease as people take enlightened charge of their own health care. The proved rules about health care are simple and easy to learn. Living by those rules, however, may require a complete change in life style for many people who have never been told much about health maintenance; and that won't be easy. Don't expect your physician to take the time to tell you about those rules during your next checkup because most physicians are not concerned with health care. They are concerned with medical services, and you need to be sick or injured or think you are sick or injured to use their medical services. Most people have never had a physician try to educate them to a healthier life style, and the cost of medical service is completely out of control and looms as a national crisis because of this failure.

In dramatic contrast to treatment by physicians, however, is the preventive-maintenance attitude of dentists. U.S. dentists lead the world in providing necessary and useful medical services that do more to maintain good health than any other medical service providers anywhere in the world. Their greatest contribution is the time and effort they take to educate patients to prevent tooth loss. It works. They provide highly individualized service at a fraction of the cost of physicians' services. A twice-yearly visit to a competent dentist for prophylaxis and repair is probably the most important financial investment anyone can make in medical service. The effectiveness of the education dentists provide patients is dramatically illustrated by the fact that we now have an over-supply of dentists. Many dental schools have closed and more are in the process of closing as more patients use regular personal and professional care, making dental repairs less necessary.

Our country is in a medical service cost crisis that has

government officials and economists deeply troubled and scrambling for a financial way out. There is an equally disturbing credibility crisis among patients that has them turning to litigation in increasing numbers, confronting failed medical practice. More and more patients are seeking alternative medical solutions as they become acutely aware of the fact that traditional methods are not working, especially in the treatment of cancer.

There seems to be an unending circle of cause and effect in medical service costs that came about after the advent of so-called health insurance. First implemented as a part of union-sought wage benefits, it seemed like a good idea when first presented. After all, it used the word "health" and that was interpreted as something everyone wanted to insure. But, except for when the benefits included dental care and sent workers for annual prophylaxis and repair, precious little health was promoted.

Instead, medical services were at the core of the benefits, and the industry saw a golden opportunity to expand business by providing all kinds of costly diagnostic testing of questionable necessity and life-prolonging support systems that threaten to bankrupt the system. Soon patients were accepting treatment that is beginning to look inhumane, just because the insurance company would pay for it. We now have hospitals with equipment and personnel that can keep people alive in a vegetative state indefinitely. If a hospital gets too crowded, patients are shunted to nursing homes for continued care. Friends and relatives are made to feel insensitive if they protest prolonging such life. Many people, afraid it might happen to them some day, are arranging for living wills that forbid life-support treatment in such cases. Families sometimes fight with government or medical service personnel about the right to allow an afflicted person to die in peace. Many are concluding that such treatment will continue so long as there is insurance money to pay the bill. When the insurance company pays only part of the charges, and relatives must make up the difference, families often face financial ruin keeping alive a patient with no hope of ever returning to a quality life.

The five-minute office call that results in a bill for sixty dollars has become commonplace because the cost is passed on to the insurance company. The patient, who usually pays only 20 percent of the total bill, is still paying the old twelve-dollar charge for the same call. The hidden charge is in the form of payments made by insurance companies, who ultimately pass the bill on to employers in premiums. Medical-insurance costs often lead all other costs of doing company business, including buying the raw materials to produce the company's product.

Attempts to curb excesses and monitor fraud brought increased record-keeping, escalating costs. As more people chose to use the insurance they were intimidated into buying, more physicians were needed, and our hospitals became flooded with physicians, many from foreign countries, some with doubtful credentials. Increased litigation, the result of a system grown too big to be personal in situations where that is essential, brought demands for still more record-keeping, along with added consultations, specialists, and higher malpractice insurance rates for practitioners.

The situation is so out of hand that many hospitals have closed their maternity wards for fear of malpractice suits. The incidence of Caesarian section births is alarmingly high as physicians try to cope with fear, hospital rules, and patient demands.

Political demands from special-interest groups push treatment close to being dangerous for medical service workers and fellow patients. Hospital budgets are strained by patients they serve who never pay their bills and the shortfall is passed along to the patients who have insurance that will pay. The insurance companies then pass the cost on to their customers through increased premiums.

Medical equipment and supply companies charge exorbitant prices and get by with it because patients seldom see their bills. Billing goes directly to insurance companies, where they are accepted without challenge when presented by a company that has many employees and a big insurance load to carry. Individual insurance purchasers, with little or no clout, often do not fair so well and suffer many more denied claims.

Drug and medical supply companies have become powerful advocates in medical schools, professional societies, and government agencies. Many people now believe they dictate medical protocol and control research. Mediocre leadership among professionals and fear of those in charge haunt and thwart physicians who would dare to question established protocol. Malpractice is defined as using a treatment method that is not in consort with accepted current medical practice. With medical supply and drug companies in the most powerful leadership positions in the medical service industry, they are able to control all new ideas and products in the industry. In turn, they control the kind of treatment for which insurance companies will pay, leaving patients without freedom of choice.

The education of physicians, of course, suffers as well. Ask any diligent medical student or concerned professor, and you will probably be appalled at their evaluation of that system. Beginning with student selection, based on the convoluted SAT testing program, the entire academic program is mired in a special brand of politics that is completely out of hand.

These are the problems that face the serious physicians with integrity and a sincere desire to help their patients and still be able to keep their positions and support their families. These are the problems that face the cancer victims who look around and see that conventional treatments are not working, but who do not know what alternatives there may be. Of course, if they do find one, their medical insurance will not cover the treatment. They stumble along with the blighted system, and many die in the process.

A brief review of modern medical treatment reveals an early reliance upon mechanics as the basis for curing all ailments. Scientists studied the skeleton, muscles, and vital organs and based all disease and treatment on these interrelating systems. They made a lot of important discoveries that enriched or saved the lives of many people. Then bacteriology and the resulting emphasis on sanitation saved even more. The discovery of penicillin and its dramatic effect on tuberculosis patients so impressed medical science that it began focusing most of its research and development on chemistry. Pharmaceutical companies flourished as drugs became and remain the accepted treatment for most ailments.

But while the drug companies were growing bigger and exerting more and more control over medical practice, a small number of physicians and scientists were independently making another revolutionary discovery, the profound effect of energy and vibrational frequencies upon the human body. In 1897 the electron was discovered by Sir J.J. Thompson, and later Sir Ernest Rutherford demonstrated that a cloud of electrons in constant motion exists surrounding the nucleus of all atoms. Albert Abrams, M.D., began to apply these discoveries to medicine, and in 1914 he wrote:

> As physicians, we dare not stand aloof from the recent progress made in science. . .the laws of physical science are universal and apply equally to living organisms and so-called inanimate things. The Electron Theory demonstrates the electrical nature of matter.
>
> In the interpretation of vital phenomena we must look deeper than the cell as revealed by the microscope. The cells constitute a super structure guided in their activity by physiochemical forces.

While the drug companies appear to refuse to recognize this hypothesis, it is the basis for Sopcak's CanCell, and it could very well hold the key to a real breakthrough in the treatment of many ailments. All individuals who are interested in their own health care should familiarize themselves with this important discovery. All members of the medical service industry should consider it required reading.

The following is a list of books recommended to get the reader started on this subject:

> *Report on Radionics* by Edward W. Russell, 1973. Neville Spearman Limited, 112 Whitfield Street, London W1P 6DP.

> *The Body Electric* by Robert O. Becker, M.D., and Gary Selden, 1985. William Morrow & Co., Inc., 105 Madison Ave., New York, NY 10016.

A New Science of Life by Rupert Sheldrake. First published in Great Britain in 1981 by Blond and Briggs, Limited. Now printed by J.P. Tarcher, Inc., Los Angeles, and distributed by Houghton Mifflin Company, Boston.

Degeneration—Regeneration by Melvin E. Page, D.D.S., 1949. Nutritional Development, 5235 Gulf Boulevard, St. Petersburg Beach, FL 33706.

Hands of Light by Barbara Ann Brennan, 1988. Bantam Books, 666 Fifth Avenue, New York, NY 10103.

A visit to any public library should supply additional titles about this fascinating subject concerning vibrational frequencies of the body cells.

The history of medicine is filled with dramatic and wonderful discoveries. Ironically, many of the people responsible for some of the most valuable contributions to medicine were severely persecuted and suffered years of ridicule before they were finally accepted. Those great medical pioneers were often vilified by ignorant, jealous members of the medical establishment. Even as cures were reported, malicious rumors were circulated, calculated to destroy anyone who dared to question the current leadership.

Dr. John Bailor III, a former editor of the *Journal of the National Cancer Institute*, and Dr. Elaine Smith of the University of Iowa Medical Center, in a special article entitled "Progress Against Cancer?" (*New England Journal of Medicine*, May 8, 1986), wrote:

> The main conclusion we draw is that some 35 years of intense effort focused largely on improving treatment must be judged a qualified failure. Results have not been what they were intended and expected to be. We think that there could be much current value in a comprehensive, consolidated, objective review of the technical reasons for this failure. What forces led to overlapping waves of interest and program emphasis, such as chemotherapy screening, virol-

ogy, immunology, and perhaps now molecular biology, that have appeared to hold more promise than they have fulfilled? Why were hopes so high, what went wrong, and can future efforts be built on more realistic expectations? Why is cancer the only major cause of death for which age-adjusted mortality rates are still increasing?

The fear of cancer and the obvious failure of accepted current treatment is looming as one of the biggest problems facing medicine today. Despite the fact that the medical service industry was unable to provide the answer, it refused to recognize its responsibility to allow a scientific investigation into Entelev, a treatment that had been used from the 1940s through the mid-1980s by patients who claim it cured them of this dread disease.

And now, CanCell, acclaimed by cured cancer patients who used it since the retirement of the Entelev Project, is being treated with the same disdain. It is long past time for a fair evaluation of this treatment. It is a time for judgment.

2
What Is Cancer?

A group of diseases or one single disease? A protein disease? Progenitor cryptocides.

The general public usually doesn't get technical about what cancer is or is not. That issue is left to the medical service industry. People are concerned with results and trust their highly paid medical consultants to deliver on demand and their medical insurance to pay the bill. Most people are content with simple explanations, believing that cancer means cells that are growing out of control, multiplying, and forming tumors. Most are able to recognize the warning signs of cancer because they get many reminders about looking for them from various government agencies and public-service organizations. If such signs are found, they are told to see their physicians and follow the accepted protocol for treatment. As the number of deaths from cancer continues to rise, however, many people are becoming concerned about the validity of that protocol. If we are to find a cure for this disease, we must first identify it for what it really is. Perhaps it is in a common misconception in this first step, identification, that lies the reason for our obvious failure to find a sure cure.

The American Cancer Society, in its *Cancer Facts and Figures—1992* (page 1), asks and gives a very simple answer to the question:

What is cancer? Cancer is a group of diseases characterized by uncontrolled growth and spread of abnormal cells. If the spread is not controlled, it can

result in death. Many cancers can be cured if detected
and treated promptly. Many others can be prevented
by life-style changes, especially avoidance of tobacco.

The National Cancer Institute (NCI) asks and answers
the same question in its latest publication, *What You Need
to Know About Cancer*, NIH Publication No. 90-1566,
Revised August 1988, Reprinted November 1989 (page 2):

> What is cancer? Cancer is really a group of dis-
> eases. There are more than 100 different types of can-
> cer, but they all are a disease of some of the body's
> cells.
> Healthy cells that make up the body's tissues grow,
> divide, and replace themselves in an orderly way.
> This process keeps the body in good repair. Some-
> times, however, normal cells lose their ability to limit
> and direct their growth. They divide too rapidly and
> grow without any order. Too much tissue is produced
> and tumors begin to form. Tumors can be either
> benign or malignant.
> Benign tumors are not cancer. They do not spread
> to other parts of the body and they are seldom a
> threat to life. Often, benign tumors can be removed
> by surgery, and they are not likely to return.
> Malignant tumors are cancer. They can invade and
> destroy nearby tissue and organs. Cancer cells also
> can spread, or metastasize, to other parts of the body,
> and form new tumors.
> Because cancer can spread, it is important for the
> doctor to find out as early as possible if a tumor is
> present and if it is cancer. As soon as a diagnosis is
> made, treatment can begin.

James Sheridan and Edward Sopcak disagree with this
popularly accepted theory of multiple cancers. They believe
that cancer is a single protein disease. They believe that all
degenerative diseases come in a fixed pattern. They explain
that normal cells are aerobic; that is, they need oxygen to
exist. Cancer, on the other hand, is an anaerobic cell—that
is, one that cannot live with oxygen—that has mutated.

Sopcak believes that the change from an aerobic to an anaerobic cell is caused by either electrical or chemical damage caused by stress that may be internal or external. He estimates that, in nine out of ten cases, anaerobic cells are formed by the lack of proper diet. He claims that electrical damage may be caused by eating oils or fats that are partially oxidized or rancid. They carry what is known as free radicals that will damage cells by lowering the fixed voltage of those cells. Equally damaging are any oils that are partly hydrogenated, such as margarine or any hardened shortening. These carry large quantities of free radicals.

Chemical damage may be done during the digestion of protein, which includes a two-phased chemical reaction. At the end of the first phase there is a chemical byproduct that is equally as damaging to the nucleic acids. Digestion of protein can be completed only if there is an adequate supply of Vitamin B6, or Pyridoxine. It is a straight-forward chemical reaction. By the age of fifty, about 75 percent of our population is deficient in B6, which occurs naturally in just about all food, including fish, vegetables, fruit, nuts and grains. However, it is fragile. If it is heated, frozen or aged, it will be destroyed. Eating fresh raw food is the best way to insure that it will remain intact.

If we continue to damage cells until they are in the electrical voltage range established by Otto Warburg (Nobel Prize winner, 1931) as being between a negative .17 and a negative .21 volts, there appears a very small bacterium that Sopcak believes the medical profession misreads as a virus. It is classified as Progenitor cryptocides, isolated by Dr. Virginia Livingston Wheeler several years ago. That bacterium aids in the transfer of the cell from being oxygen-using, or aerobic, to being anaerobic, or in a state of fermentation.

Fermentation cells change the form of energy production in the body. Oxygen-using cells create their energy in the form of ATP, the chemical which stores energy. Anaerobic cells also end up with ATP, but with a different quantity of it; the body recognizes the change in the creation of energy and tends to protect itself by the deposition of abnormal protein. All of the protein or collagen diseases occur at that point. Depending upon the genetics of the body, there will be malfunction or diseases such as lupis, late-onset diabetes, muscular dystrophy, multiple sclerosis, scleroderma, etc.

If there is a chronic demand (and it must be a chronic demand) on the cell structure for energy that is in excess of what that cell structure is programmed to deliver, the body answers that demand for energy with the mutation of the anaerobic cell. All cancer is a mutated anaerobic cell, and that is an irreversible condition.

Some researchers are attempting to reverse the anaerobic cell and turn it back into an aerobic cell by the use of nutrients or oxygen and other methods. Sheridan and Sopcak believe it cannot be done; it is irreversible. Both Entelev and CanCell take the anaerobic cell, which is already in low voltage, and lower the voltage further. Recognizing the respiratory cycle of that cell, an electrical blockage is created, taking the voltage past the primitive stage back to the building-block stage where the hydrogen bond joining the coils of the protein helix is shifted. When this is done, the anaerobic cancer cell will lyse, or self-digest. It changes from cancer to a waste material, composed of two amino acids that have the appearance of raw egg whites, which the body eliminates any way it can. It may appear in the urine or the stool or as a vaginal discharge. It may be vomited or coughed up, and it may be eliminated in perspiration. The cancer cells are subsequently replaced with normal oxygen-using cells.

That is a very simple explanation of the cancer-cell hypothesis upon which Entelev and CanCell were developed. You will find in Chapter 5 (Document No. 8) a reprint of Sheridan's *Technology of Entelev, IND-20258*, which was printed and distributed free of charge to anyone who cared to read it, reprint it, and pass it on to others. On page 21 of that pamphlet is his explanation of carcinogenesis, how cancer is formed, in scientific detail. It gives a thorough understanding of this hypothesis, which is a radical departure from the accepted theory of the American Cancer Society and the NCI.

In 1990, Phillip W. Maly, O.D., wrote an explanation of the protein theory entitled *Cancer: A Protein Disease* from information he obtained from Sheridan. It too was printed and widely copied and circulated in the same manner, free of charge for anyone to read, copy, and pass on to others. It is included here in its entirety. See Document No. 1, page 29.

A note should be added here concerning Progenitor cryptocides, around which there is a great deal of controversy. Dr. Livingston Wheeler's Clinic in San Diego, California, treated cancer patients there with a complex unorthodox therapy that prompted investigation by the American Cancer Society. Based on their files as of February 1989, the ACS printed an article entitled "Livingston-Wheeler Therapy" (*CA-A Cancer Journal For Clinicians*, Vol. 40, No. 2, March/April 1990) that included the following:

> Summary:
> Livingston-Wheeler's cancer treatment is based on the belief that cancer is caused by a bacterium she has named Progenitor cryptocides. Careful research using modern techniques, however, has shown that there is no such organism and that Livingston-Wheeler has apparently mistaken several different types of bacteria, both rare and common, for a unique microbe. In spite of diligent research to isolate a cancer-causing microorganism, none has been found. . .

This ACS opinion is disputed by a number of respected professionals and is another theory that could and should be settled by competent unbiased research.

CANCER: A PROTEIN DISEASE

Written by Phillip W. Maly O.D.,
from information obtained from J. Sheridan

May 4, 1990

INTRODUCTION

This is an introduction to the concept of cancer as a "protein disease". The disease process is one of abnormal cellular respiration and energy transfer resulting in less differentiated (more primitive) protein molecule formation. (i.e., in cancer the proteins of normally differentiated cells become less differentiated, thereby changing cellular structure and function.)

It is being suggested here that a protein disease is caused by a shift (a slight increase) in the energy level of the hydrogen bonds joining the successive coils of the protein helix. The increase in the hydrogen bond energy level produces a greater separation between the turns of the helix and, if large enough, a resultant loss of differentiation.

Where does the energy for the hydrogen bonds come from? To answer this question, let us first digress to the energy cycle of nature.

Refer to Figure A, THE ENERGY CYCLE OF NATURE.

Reviewing what happens when photosynthesis occurs:

Energy in the form of light strikes a leaf.

OH^- breaks up.

O_2 is given off.

Energy units ($ee-H^+$) - go down the redox scale.

Glucose is manufactured.

The reverse occurs in the human body:

Glucose is broken down.

A variable portion of the units go up the redox scale transferring their protential energy (voltage) to form ATP along the way.

1

O_2 is picked up.

OH^- is given off ... and the cycle is completed.

The remainder of the units that do not go up the redox scale are retained in chemical structures such as lactic acid and amino acids to be used, in part, as the energy for the hydrogen bonds.

Protein disease is defined in terms of two energy units, ATP and $(ee\text{-}H^+)\text{-}$, and is the relative ratio of:

    A.   The number of ATP molecules being formed (at the expense of energy derived from $(ee\text{-}H^+)^-$ units.)

    to   The number of high energy $(ee\text{-}H^+)^-$ units remaining in chemical structures to serve, among other things, as hydrogen bonds.

    B.   Note: The $(ee\text{-}H^+)^-$ unit is normally' symbolized as H^-; the hybride ion. The $(eeH^+)^-$ symbol is used here to emphasize the presence of the two electrons which carry the energy.

           The energy of the two electron units is of particular importance because, among other things, it is the energy of the hydrogen bond.

           A glucose molecule has the capacity to form 12 $(eeH^+)^-$ units which, in turn, have the capacity to form 36 ATP molecules.

The part played by ATP energy in protein formation is relatively clear. The ATP provides the energy to join a pool of individual amino acids into a chain of amino acids.

The $(eeH^+)^-$ unit, however, is much more versatile:

2

In normal cellular respiration, the 12 $(ee^+H)^-$ from a glucose molecule provide 100% of the energy to make ATP.

In a primitive cell, only about 5% of the $(ee^+H)^-$ units are used to form ATP; and, about 95% become a part of lactic acid.

This can be illustrated by hypothetical events in a model cell where:

Cell 1 (Normal)   A single glucose molecule goes through the normal repiratory pathway to form 36 ATP molecules.

Cell 2 (Primitive)   A single glucose molecule goes through glycolysis to form 2 lactic acid molecules and 2 ATP Molecules.

Cell 3 (Cancer)   A single glucose molecule goes through the respiratory pathway to form 24 ATP molecules while 6 glucose molecules go through glycolysis to form 12 ATP molecules and 12 lactic acid molecules.

Refer again to Figure A.

The left side of the diagram shows the step-wise oxidation of glucose via the respiratory system wherein the energy from each $(ee^-H^+)^-$ unit in the glucose structure is used to form 3 ATP molecules.

Potentially, the 12 $(ee^-H^+)^-$ units form 12 of the ATP molecules going up the left side of Figure A could form a total of 36 ATP molecules. Of special interest here is that the 12 $(ee^-H^+)^-$ units form 12 of the ATP molecules in the energy jump from cytochrome b to cytochrome c in a normal cell. However, this does not occur in a cancer cell.

It beomes apparent that if every molecule of glucose in the model is oxidized by proceeding along the left side of the diagrom, 100% of the $(ee^-H^+)^-$ energy would be consumed in forming 36 ATP molecules and there would be no energy remaining to form hydrogen bonds.

3

Left Side

ATP energy derived from (ee-H+)- energy   100.0%

(ee-H+)- energy remaining   0.0%

However, if every molecule of glucose in the model went along the right side of the diagram, there would be 2 molecules of ATP formed at a cost of about 5% of the (ee-H+)- energy.

Right Side

ATP energy derived from (ee-H+)- energy   about 5%

(ee-H+)- energy remaining   about 95%

Query: Returning to the left side of Figure A, what could be expected to happen if an outside influence would prevent 12 of the 36 ATP molecules from forming - as would occur if the (ee-H+)- jump from cytochrome b to cytochrome c would stop forming 12 ATP molecules.

Answer: One could expect that there would be an increase in ATP production on the right side of Figure A; that is, produce the missing 12 ATP molecules.

Totals
(From the 7 Glucose Molecules)

ATP molecules   about 14%
(ee-H+)- units remaining   about 18%

These percentages are characteristic of cancer tissue.

The sevenfold increase in the metabolic rate of glucose metabolism is also characteristic of cancer tissue.

Figure B illustrates the above.

4

The left edge of Figure B shows the energy relationship on the left side of Figure A. The Y is the percent conversion (100%) of $(ee^-H^+)^-$ energy to ATP and the X is the percentage (0.0) of $(ee^-H^+)^-$ remaining in the chemical structures.

The right edge of Figure B shows Y at about 5% and X at about 95% - a primitive cell picture.

The "cancer picture" shows Y at about 14% and X at about 86%. This suggests that carcinogenesis is a shift in the nature of the energy supply toward the primitive with the shift being interrupted at the steady state of cancer.

Also illustrated is the elongation of the helical protein structure due to the increased energy of the hydrogen bond.

> In a normal cell having a normal relationship of X to Y, the production of ATP varies with the work demand to maintain a steady state. Within the normal work demand range, relatively constant spacing between the coils of the helix is maintained and only minor changes occur.
>
> However, in the cancer relationship, the increase in the hydrogen bond energy level produces a substantial increase in the coil spacing. The increased elongation is sufficient to prevent the replication of normal protein.
>
> At or near the primitive relationship, still greater elongation prevents even the cancer protein helix from replicating itself. With the production of even aberrant protein impossible, the cell lyses.

Treatment

The figures suggest and research has shown that cancer can be treated by causing the additional shift in the energy supply toward the primitive steady state where glycolysis would be the sole source of energy to the cell.

This is done by a system of compounds having redox systems which mimic those of respiratory enzymes. The compounds can to some extent block $(ee^-H^+)^-$ flow through the asceding redox levels, and to some extent shunt $(ee^-H^+)^-$ directly to oxygen, the terminal acceptor, and out of the system.

COMMENTS

CANCELL, DEVELOPED BY J. SHERIDAN, IS SUCH A SYSTEM OF COMPOUNDS THAT MIMIC THE RESPIRATORY ENZYMES.

CANCELL:

IS NON-TOXIC.

HAS NO KNOWN ADVERSE SIDE EFFECTS EXCEPT TEMPORARY, MODERATE FATIGUE.

WILL EFFECTIVELY TREAT 80% OF RANDOMLY SELECTED CANCER PATIENTS.
EFFECTIVELY TREAT MEANS NO CLINICAL SIGNS OR SYMPTOMS OF ACTIVE DISEASE.

WILL EFFECTIVELY TREAT OVER 90% OF COLLAGEN DISEASE PATIENTS.

6

FIGURE A:
THE ENERGY CYCLE OF NATURE

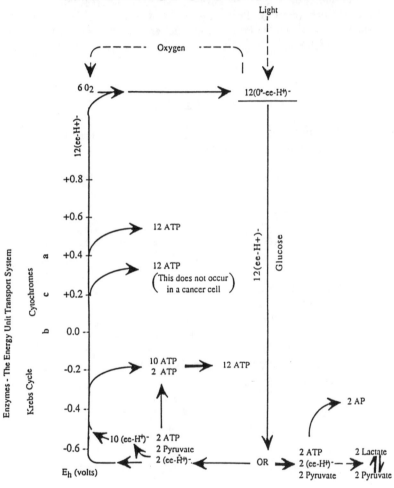

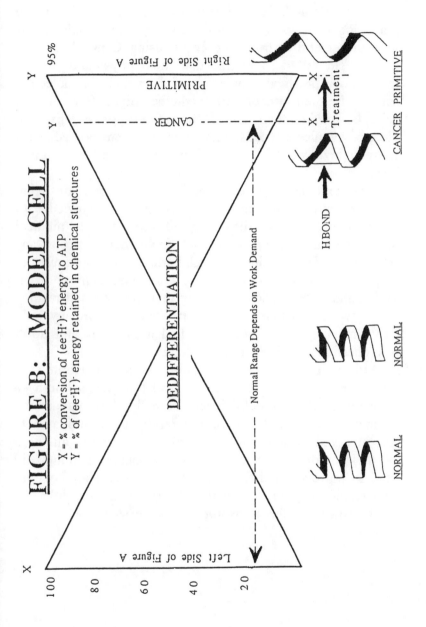

FIGURE B: MODEL CELL

X = % conversion of (ee·H·)· energy to ATP
Y = % of (ee·H·)· energy retained in chemical structures

DEDIFFERENTIATION

Normal Range Depends on Work Demand

Left Side of Figure A

Right Side of Figure A

PRIMITIVE

CANCER

HBOND

Treatment

NORMAL   NORMAL   CANCER   PRIMITIVE

95%

100
80
60
40
20

Dr. Maly wrote his treatise attempting to explain cellular respiration in simple language that medical professionals could understand. He believed that, if he could educate practicing physicians around the country, they would recognize the scientific truth and begin using CanCell to treat cancer. He failed to realize that most physicians do not make much practical application of their study of molecular science in their practice of medicine. Since few medical schools teach much about the effects of energy and electrodynamics on cells, they probably were not educated to recognize what he was talking about and so ignored him.

After graduating, most physicians enter the mainstream of their limited environments, shelving their knowledge of basic science along with their old textbooks. Is medical school so intimidating as to shut down their curiosity and dedication? Is it medical school burnout, peer pressure, or fear of governing authorities that halts their clinical observation and investigation? Limiting their professional reading to a few establishment and pharmaceutical company publications, they trust those so-called authorities and don't ask questions, at least not out loud.

Although hundreds of copies were distributed to physicians, few took the time to read this treatise from an unrecognized, non-establishment Nobody. Few understood it, and those who did were apparently too intimidated to get involved with using it or bringing it to the attention of their medical peers. Hundreds of cancer patients did read it, however, and thought it made sense. They couldn't understand why the medical industrial complex didn't at least investigate the possibilities it suggested.

3
The Big Three Names
Associated With Cancer

*The American Cancer Society (ACS). The National
Cancer Institute (NCI). The Food and Drug
Administration (FDA). Traditional treatment vs.
Entelev/CanCell.*

Most people would be surprised, maybe even shocked,
to learn that there is no nationwide cancer registry. There
is no way of knowing exactly how many new cases of
cancer are diagnosed in the U.S. every year. The ACS, in
"Sources of Statistics" in its *Cancer Facts and Figures—
1992*, explains that it uses the NCI's Surveillance, Epidemiology and End Results (SEER) program to evaluate cancer
trends. The ACS estimates of U.S. cancer cases diagnosed
in 1992 are reported to be based on age-specific incidence
rates from the SEER program for 1986-1988, applied to
the 1992 Census population projections, adjusted to accom-
modate sites with recently increasing or decreasing rates.
With all of today's sophisticated computer capability, this
kind of record-keeping must be considered a national dis-
grace.

There are three organizations that influence or control,
directly or indirectly, the study of the causes and treatment
of cancer. Of course, there are people all over the world
who are doing all kinds of independent research, but they
must ultimately deal with at least one of these organizations
to begin to have their findings tested and substantiated
before being sanctioned to be made available to patients
in the U.S.

The American Cancer Society

The American Cancer Society is undoubtedly the best-known entity associated with cancer, thanks mostly to its yearly fund-raising campaigns. It is a voluntary organization founded in New York City in 1913 by a group of ten physicians and five laymen who called it the American Society for the Control of Cancer. The name was later changed to the American Cancer Society, and it is now one of the largest voluntary health-related organizations in the U.S. It is composed of fifty-seven incorporated chartered divisions (one in each state, Puerto Rico, the District of Columbia, and five metropolitan areas), and there are 3,300 local units. The divisions are represented by a 206-member House of Delegates, and there is additional representation based on population. A 124-member elected, voting Board of Directors sets policy for the Society. State programs are planned by division and unit boards of directors. Priorities and goals are developed by departments of Research, Detection and Treatment, Prevention, Public Information, Communications, Epidemiology and Statistics, Patient Services, Advocacy, and Income Development.

The Society may be contacted at:

National Headquarters
American Cancer Society
1599 Clifton Road N. E.
Atlanta, GA 30329-4251
Phone: 800-227-2345

The information provided here is taken from *Cancer Facts & Figures—1992*, a thirty-page publication the ACS provides free for the asking.

In the 1990 Annual Report, the ACS reported a total budget for 1990-91 of $367,793,000, allocated as follows:

Fund-raising	(16%)	58,847,000
Prevention	(19%)	69,881,000
Research	(26.2%)	96,362,000

Community Services	(7.3%)	26,849,000
Patient Services	(13.8%)	51,122,000
Management & General	(7.2%)	26,481,000
Detection & Treatment	(10.4%)	38,251,000

The ACS to date has invested more than $1.4 billion ($1,400,000,000) in cancer research, growing from $1 million in 1946 to $94 million in 1991. The Research Program budget includes five major types of grants:

1. Research and Clinical Investigation Grants (about 75%) to finance specific research projects;

2. Research Personnel Grants (18%+) to provide salary support for established scientists and postdoctoral fellows specializing in cancer research;

3. Institutional Research Grants to universities, institutes and hospitals to support pilot studies by new investigators;

4. Research Development Program Grants to provide rapid funding for priority projects; and

5. Special Institutional Grants to provide long-term funding for interdisciplinary projects.

The ACS reports that cancer is treated by surgery, radiation, radioactive substances, chemicals, hormones, and immunotherapy. It reports that trends in diagnosis and treatment in the 1990s include four areas:

1. Genetic Engineering, potentially using powerful new drugs, correcting impaired immune systems, and modifying heredity by transplanting foreign genes. They identify as promising TNF, the tumor necrosis factor; interleukin-2; and certain bone-marrow growth-regulators.

2. Monoclonal Antibodies that will preferentially

recognize cancer cells, providing early detection. Claims are made that monoclonal antibodies already have been used to deliver drugs directly to tumors, killing them but sparing healthy tissue.

3. Mechanisms of carcinogenesis that investigate cancer development in humans.

4. Chemoprevention including the use of vitamin A, retinoids, vitamins C and E, selenium, and natural-ly-occurring substances found in foodstuffs.

The National Cancer Institute

The National Cancer Institute is one of sixteen research institutes that are part of the National Institutes of Health, which are part of the Department of Health and Human Services, along with the Public Health Service. It is the federal government's principal agency for research on cancer causes, prevention, diagnosis, treatment, rehabilitation, and information about cancer. It sports a low profile compared to the ACS, and few people have ever heard of it. The NCI publishes a long list of free publications which may be ordered from a publications list available by calling or writing their office.

The NCI is funded by annual appropriations from Congress and supports research at headquarters in Bethesda, Maryland, and in laboratories and medical centers throughout the U.S. and the rest of the world. The 1992 budget was for $746,035,000. The Institute may be contacted at:

National Cancer Institute
9000 Rockville Pike
Bethesda, MD 20892
Phone: 301-496-4000 (National Institutes of Health)

In the pamphlet *What You Need to Know About Cancer*, which is provided free of charge upon request, the NCI lists five methods of treating cancer with a brief explanation of each, which are summarized here:

1. Surgery is a local treatment that removes the tumor and any nearby tissue that may contain cancer cells. Cancer cells can travel through the bloodstream or lymphatic system, so doctors often remove lymph nodes that are near the tumor to see if they contain cancer cells. Side effects may be numbness or tingling in the area when nerves may be cut during surgery. These problems usually go away within a few weeks, although some numbness may be permanent.

2. Radiation therapy (also called x-ray therapy, radiotherapy, cobalt treatment, or irradiation) is a local treatment that uses high-energy rays to damage cancer cells so they are unable to grow and multiply. For some cancers, like leukemia and lymphoma, the whole body may be radiated. The two most common types of radiation therapy are external and implants. In external radiation therapy, a machine directs high-energy rays at the cancer. Patients receiving external radiation therapy are not radioactive during or after treatment. In implants, a small container of radioactive material is placed in the body cavity or directly into the cancer. The patient must remain hospitalized while the implant is in place and the material may transmit rays into the area around the patient, so visits and contacts with these patients are limited during treatment. Side effects may include unusual tiredness, skin reactions in the area being treated, and a decrease in the number of white blood cells, which help to protect the body against infection.

3. Chemotherapy is a systemic treatment that uses anticancer drugs to destroy cancer cells. There are many different kinds of drugs, and they may be given by mouth or injected into a muscle, vein, or artery. Chemotherapy works mainly on cancer cells, but also affects other rapidly growing cells, including hair cells and cells that line the digestive tract. Side effects include hair loss, nausea, and vomiting. Most anticancer drugs also affect the bone marrow, decreasing its ability to produce blood cells, presenting a higher risk of getting an infection.

4. Hormone therapy uses drugs to block the body's production of hormones or surgery to remove hormone-producing organs to treat the types of cancer that depend on hormones for their growth. Commonly used drugs include tamoxifen (for breast cancer), DES or diethylstilbestrol (for breast and prostate cancers), and Megace (for kidney and uterine cancers). Side effects include nausea and vomiting, swelling, or weight gain. In some cases the treatment interferes with the body's production or use of hormones (for example, tamoxifen sometimes induces symptoms of menopause).

5. Biological therapy, sometimes called immunotherapy, tries to boost the body's immune system to fight the cancer. One form uses monoclonal antibodies to locate cancer cells and bind to them; another uses interferon to stimulate the body's immune system; and a third uses interleukin-2, a protein that regulates cell growth.

The Food and Drug Administration

The Food and Drug Administration is a federal regulatory agency charged with enforcing the Federal Food, Drug and Cosmetic Act and several related public-health laws, including those governing the nation's blood supply. It employs some 1,100 investigators and inspectors to cover the country's more than 90,000 FDA-regulated businesses. There are district and local offices in 157 cities across the country. The agency may be contacted at:

U.S. Food and Drug Administration
5600 Fishers Lane
Rockville, MD 20857
Phone: 800-231-3280

FDA investigators and inspectors reportedly visit more than 20,000 facilities a year and collect more than 70,000 domestic and imported product samples for examination by FDA scientists or for label checks. The agency employs

2,100 scientists, including 900 chemists and 300 microbiologists who work in forty laboratories in the Washington, D.C., area and around the country. Some of these scientists analyze samples and others review test results submitted by companies seeking agency approval for drugs, vaccines, food additives, coloring agents and medical devices.

The FDA operates the National Center for Toxicological Research in Jefferson, Arkansas, which investigates the biological effects of widely used chemicals, and the Engineering and Analytical Center in Winchester, Massachusetts, which tests medical devices, radiation-emitting products, and radioactive drugs.

In deciding whether to approve new drugs, the FDA does not itself do research, but rather examines the results of studies done by the manufacturer. The agency must determine that a new drug produces the benefits it is supposed to without causing side effects that would outweigh those benefits.

All three of these organizations are aware of CanCell and have become involved with it at some time or other.

The American Cancer Society provides a rather lengthy printout on the subject, free of charge upon request, identifying the source of the material as coming from their ACS Questionable Methods of Cancer Management, 1991, filed on computer views 8202 through 8206. A re-typed copy is printed here, as Document No. 2:

American Cancer Society
Cancer Response System
Printed On: 12/16/91
CANCELL/ENTELEV

After study of the literature and other available information, the American Cancer Society has found no evidence that the use of Cancell/Entelev results in objective benefit in the treatment of cancer in human beings. Lacking such evidence, the American Cancer

Society strongly urges individuals with cancer not to seek treatment from practitioners utilizing this compound.

The following is a summary of material on Cancell, also known as Entelev, Jim's Juice, Crocinic Acid, Sheridan's Formula, JS-114, JS-101, and 126-F, on file with the American Cancer Society as of June 1991. No implication of agreement by the Society with the contents of any proponent material is to be construed because of the Society's reference to that material.

BACKGROUND

Cancell or Entelev is the name given to a nostrum being touted as a cure for all forms of cancer and a wide variety of other diseases.

The substance was first envisioned in 1936 by James V. Sheridan, a chemist working at the time for Dow Chemical. According to a 1984 magazine interview with Sheridan, the idea for Entelev came to him in a dream that he believes was inspired by God.

Because Entelev was divinely inspired, Sheridan says, he felt that he could not charge desperate people for its use. Therefore, he provided it free to patients with serious forms of cancer.

By 1953, Sheridan claims, his product was ready for clinical trials, but because he could not provide the American Cancer Society with adequate proof that he "owned the idea," no trials were held. (He still incorrectly believes that the Society somehow controls clinical trials.) Sheridan also claims that because of this he was fired from his job at the Detroit Institute of Cancer Research. Since then, he has persisted in his development of Entelev and in treating cancer patients.

In 1982, Sheridan requested that the United States Food and Drug Administration (FDA) give Entelev status as an investigational new drug. Although the preparation was assigned an investigational new drug number (IND #20258), the FDA requested additional information prior to allowing clinical testing in humans to proceed. As of the date of this publication, the IND remains inactive, because appropriate information regarding the chemical makeup of Entelev and studies showing its efficacy in animal models have not been provided to the FDA.

In 1984, Sheridan claims that he was forced by the media and the FDA to stop manufacturing Entelev. At that point, a second promoter, Edward J.Sopcak, acquired the directions for its manufacture from Sheridan and began providing it to patients under the name Cancell, which is his registered trademark. Like Sheridan, Sopcak provides his product free of charge to seriously ill patients with cancer and AIDS. According to available information, the promoters absorb the cost of its manufacture.

In February 1989, the FDA asked for and received a permanent injunction against Sheridan and Sopcak prohibiting them or their agents from introducing Entelev/Cancell or their components into interstate commerce on the basis that they were adulterated, misbranded, and unapproved new drugs. Sopcak points out, however, that the injunction does not prevent him "from making a gift of Cancell to anyone in the world who requests it," so he has continued its manufacture and distribution.

PROMOTIAL [sic] CLAIMS

Sheridan's role in the promotion of Cancell/Entelev has been superseded by that of Edward J. Sopcak. Although literature Sopcak provides says that "no claims are made for Cancell," he regularly promotes it as a cure for many diseases, including cancer, AIDS, collagen disease, lupus, scleroderma, cystic fibrosis, multiple sclerosis, adult-onset diabetes mellitus, mental illness (except schizophrenia), emphysema, Parkinson's disease, hemophilia, hypo- and hypertension, and some forms of epilepsy. For most of these conditions, he says, cure is very rapid. In the case of epilepsy, for example, seizures are claimed to be reduced by 50 percent within five seconds of taking the compound. Sopcak also claims that Cancell protects against radiation. Although the FDA has prohibited the manufacture and interstate shipment of Cancell, claiming that it is an unapproved new drug, Sopcak claims that it is not a drug, but rather "an assembly of synthetic chemicals" that react with the body electrically rather than chemically.

The promoters claim that 80 percent of randomly selected cancer patients who take Cancell are "effectively treated" (defined as the patient being left with no clinical signs of disease) and that the product is nontoxic and has no side effects. The promoters say that their claims are based on experiments with tens of thousands of test animals and about 20,000 humans. Furthermore, according to Sopcak, benefits are seen with Cancell even though three out of four of the people who take Cancell have been deemed terminal and beyond orthodox medical help.

RATIONALE

The rationale for the mechanism of Cancell/Entelev and its use against cancer are provided by Sheridan in two pamphlets, "Cancer: A Protein Disease," and "The Technology of Entelev, IND-20258 and Cancell, an Identical Material." According to Sheridan, cancer is a protein disease. There are, he says, three types of cells: normal, primitive, and cancer (malignant) cells. He states that in the "cancer relationship" (when an individual has cancer rather than normal cells), cellular proteins become less differentiated than usual and can replicate only cancer proteins. The function of Cancell/Entelev, according to Sheridan, is to cause cells to attain the "primitive state." In this condition, he claims, the cells will self-destruct.

Sopcak's description of the etiology of cancer and Cancell's mode of action is somewhat different from that of Sheridan's. Sopcak claims that there is only one type of cancer and that it is caused by a mutated anaerobic cell. Lack of proper diet is the culprit, causing electrical and chemical damage, he says. "Progenitor cryptocides" (a microorganism described by Virginia Livingston-Wheeler) becomes active and helps cause healthy cells to respire anaerobically, he says. When the demand for energy exceeds the anaerobic cell's ability to produce it, the cell mutates and becomes a cancer cell, he says. This state, according to Sopcak, is irreversible. Cancell acts, by changing the vibrational frequency and energy of cancer cells until they reach the "primitive state" described by Sheridan. This causes them to self-digest, Sopcak says. The cellular waste material, which "has the appearance of raw egg whites" then passes out of the body any way it can—in the urine, in the stool, as a vaginal discharge, or in perspiration, or is thrown up or coughed up. The cancer cells are then claimed to be replaced with normal healthy cells. Sopcak believes that in the future all medicine will be practiced by adjusting vibrational frequencies.

THE CANCELL/ENTELEV FORMULATION

Batches of Cancell/Entelev are manufactured by its promoters in their homes. In the FDA's February 1989 complaint, the agency itemized the ingredients of Cancell/Entelev as inositol, nitric acid, sodium sulfite, potassium hydroxide, sulfuric acid, and catechol. Sheridan has stated that he also uses crocinic acid. These ingredients are heated for the better part of a day (four batches in an eight-hour cycle), resulting in batches of dark brown liquid that fill 25 pint bottles, which are then refrigerated. The identities of the compounds produced by this procedure are somewhat uncertain.

Dr. Tadeusz Malinski, an Associate Professor of Analytical Chemistry at Oakland University in Rochester, Michigan, working under a small grant from the Eden Foundation, a nonprofit corporation created by Sheridan and Sopcak, has spent considerable time trying to analyze the components of the final Cancell/Entelev formulation. Dr. Malinski has succeeded in identifying a minimum of 12 different compounds, none of which are known to be effective for curing any forms of cancer.

Sopcak claims that once he prepares the formula, he "tunes" it so it has the correct vibrational frequency to work properly. He fails to describe, however, how such tuning is accomplished. Sheridan says that he is still modifying his formulation to make it more effective.

THE CANCELL/ENTELEV REGIMEN

Cancell is a liquid recommended for both internal and external use. Sopcak recommends that it be administered by both of these routes simultaneously for the best results. The regimen lasts for 45 days or until all signs of the disease are gone. According to proponents, the patient must not smoke during the treatment, since nicotine prevents Cancell from working by inhibiting the immune system. Vitamins also should not be taken, because they raise the energy of the cell, while Cancell lowers it, the proponents say.

Finally, the promoters discourage patients from using Cancell with any other cancer therapy.

INTERNAL USE

Cancell may be administered either orally or rectally. Orally, one fourth of a teaspoon is held under the tongue for five minutes and then swallowed. This is said to enable sublingual absorption of a portion of the dosage. The procedure and dosage must be repeated every six hours, night and day. Rectally one fourth of a teaspoon may be injected into the rectum with a plastic medicine dropper every six hours.

EXTERNAL USE

For external usage, an area on the inside of the wrist or ball of the foot is thoroughly cleaned with soap and water. The area is then dampened with several drops of dimethylsulfoxide (DMSO). Cancell/Entelev is then placed on a quilted cotton pad and taped onto the treated area.

ADJUVANT THERAPY

Along with the internal and external applications of Cancell, Sopcak recommends 1,000mg doses of bromelain, a digestive aid, before each meal. If Cancell is taken for AIDS, the patient is also supposed to take at least 1,000mg of glutathione before each meal. Additionally, patients with AIDS, herpes, or Epstein-Barr virus are advised to take 2,000mg of butylated hydroxytoluene before retiring each night.

COST

As previously discussed, neither promoter charges for his product. Sopcak and Sheridan have, however, founded the Eden Foundation, a nonprofit corporation. Patients who so desire may make contributions to the foundation. According to Sheridan, the donations are used to help offset the cost of the manufacture of Cancell/Entelev and to fund research. According to an FDA spokesman, the Eden Foundation receives only a small number of donations.

EVALUATION

As is the case with many questionable "cancer cures," serious questions are raised about the scientific rationale for the use of Cancell/Entelev. Sheridan's basic physiological model is neither logical, nor in keeping with contemporary knowledge of cell structure and physiology or the etiology of cancer. Likewise, the claim that all cancers are a single disease with a common cause is archaic.

Sheridan's contention that cells exist in one of three states—primitive, differentiated, or malignant—is, by his own acknowledgment, simplistic. Obviously there are hundreds of different cell types with various structures, functions, and metabolic requirements. Moreover there are respiratory metabolic pathways other than those considered by Sheridan that would have to be considered in any discussion of respiratory energetics.

The promoters' thesis is that normal cells placed under chronic energy stress mutate and become malignant by reaching a metabolic "steady state" where they integrate aerobic and anaerobic respiratory pathways in a irreversible and abnormal manner. Such cells, Sheridan claims, have voltages (redox potentials) that are lower than normal. Sheridan is unable to provide any data demonstrating the consistent potential changes or voltage measurements that he claims are characteristic of malignancies. Furthermore, the contemporary body of peer-reviewed literature describes no such process or pattern of abnormalities. Nor is evidence provided that cancer is caused when respiration is "damaged" by the uncoupling of the electron transport system from phosphorylation.

Sheridan claims that his theory supports and explains Nobel laureate Otto Warburg's observation that cancer cells have relatively high anaerobic respiration rates. Modern researchers, however, attribute the increased anaerobic respiration rate in some tumors to lack of oxygen in poorly vascularized tissue surrounding rapidly growing tumors rather than, as claimed by Sheridan, to an inherent inability of cancer cells to utilize oxygen.

Cancell/Entelev is purported to cure cancer by reducing the voltage of cancer cells until they become "primitive." Because the energy not utilized in respiration energizes helical proteins, Cancell/Entelev supposedly causes the destruction of the hydrogen bonds holding the coils in place. This is said to happen because Cancell/Entelev blocks mitochondrial electron transport. When asked why normal cells are not equally affected, Sheridan replies that they are but that their voltages are not lowered chronically or low enough to cause them to become malignant or die. This explanation, however, is not in keeping with the known effects of other electron transport inhibitors such as sodium azide, which, if ingested, can result in death.

To date, no deaths from Cancell/Entelev have been reported to the FDA or in the peer-reviewed literature. Thus, it appears that the formulation either does not act as postulated by Sheridan, or that the doses are so minute that potential problems are not evident. Sheridan does point out, however, that patients may experience "temporary, moderate fatigue" after taking Cancell/Entelev. No mention is made of other symptoms that might be associated with respiratory distress.

The promoters claim that Cancell has been tested on thousands of test animals and humans (Sopcak alone claims to have manufactured and distributed about 15,000 pints to patients), and that it is safe and effective in treating 80 percent of randomly selected cancer patients. Sopcak, although claiming that there have been no double-blind clinical trials, says that the FDA did a "secret and illegal" study and determined that 80 to 85 percent of cancer patients had no malignant cells left in their bodies after treatment. According to FDA spokesman Kenneth Shelin, however, no such study was ever conducted.

In 1978 and 1980, the National Cancer Institute (NCI) conducted animal tests on Entelev (JS-101) provided by Sheridan and determined that it had no significant anticancer activity and did not warrant further study.

In the fall of 1990 and again in the winter of 1991, the NCI examined samples of Cancell under the Institute's "In Vitro Anticancer Drug Discovery Program." Based on the negative results obtained under their current screening procedures the Screening Data Review Committee state that the "NCI has determined that no further action will be taken on this compound."

Sheridan claims that many other studies have been performed demonstrating the benefits of Cancell/Entelev, but because the results were favorable, he says, the work was suppressed by "The Establishment." Sopcak also states that the FDA and pharmaceutical companies are working to suppress positive results because they have a vested interest in the "cancer treatment industry."

In reality, the only evidence that Sheridan and Sopcak have to offer is testimonial. Sopcak states that he has a file of over a thousand letters, many with documentation, that say Cancell works, but that no clinical trials have been done. Wendland found Sheridan's evidence to be "ridiculous and amateurish."

Although the promoters claim their product is highly effective against all cancers and against a wide variety of other diseases including AIDS, no reasonable body of peer-review literature exists that would substantiate their claims. Not only is the basic rationale behind the theoretical mode of action of Cancell/Entelev scientifically unsound, but it has not been tested for safety or efficacy.

Cancell/Entelev is not produced in conformity with

good manufacturing practices and is considered by the FDA to be adulterated, misbranded, and inadequately labeled. The composition and potency may vary from batch to batch, and bottles fail to carry appropriate warnings or adequate directions for its use.

Perhaps the most serious danger from using Cancell/Entelev, however, is Sopcak's insistence that patients abandon other forms of cancer therapy when using their product. Thus, patients who might respond well to proven methods of cancer control miss the opportunity to be helped by responsible practitioners.

RECOMMENDATIONS

There is no evidence that Cancell/Entelev will cure cancer or other degenerative diseases. The American Cancer Society, therefore, strongly urges individuals with cancer not to seek treatment with this product.

SOURCE: ACS Questionable Methods of Cancer Management, 1991.

Unlike the swift and thorough cooperation by the ACS that resulted in the production of their evaluation of Can-Cell/Entelev by return mail, repeated calls to the NCI asking for information about Entelev/CanCell have resulted in negative responses that must be called the epitome of buck-passing. Upon calling the published National Institutes of Health phone number, 301-496-400, I was referred to no less than six other phone numbers and finally told that if I wanted any information I would have to get it by application to the Freedom of Information Staff, HFI-35, Food and Drug Administration, 5600 Fishers Lane, Rockville, Maryland 20857.

Meanwhile, documents given to me by Edward Sopcak indicate that the NCI has screened preparations presented by James Sheridan on at least two occasions. A letter from Ven L. Narayanan, Ph.D., dated October 2, 1990, refers to a prior screening of a Sheridan preparation, JS-101, and states, "The compound was determined to be inactive," but asks for a new testing. (See Document No. 3, page 57.)

James Sheridan's October 15, 1990, reply indicates that he sent the sample requested and calls attention to the fact that errors were committed during the first testing. (See Document No. 4, page 58.) In a phone call, he explained that the errors were in the time allotted for the testing. He explained that the NCI followed an established regimen of allowing the same specific time for all tests and that his preparation needed a different specified, specific time to be effective.

A follow-up letter from Michael R. Boyd, M.D., Ph.D., dated December 21, 1990, contains NCI in-vitro testing results that indicate negative growth results in each of the CanCell tests conducted. However, no indication of any further pending action by NCI was included, despite the letter's reference to that in paragraph three. (See Document No. 5, page 59.)

A call to the Food and Drug Administration in December 1992 resulted in my being told that agency had recently filed action in federal court in Michigan and won an injunction to prevent Mr. Sopcak from further making or distributing CanCell. I asked for a written summary of the petition and verdict. I was told that they didn't have one and that I would need to purchase a transcript of the trial from the court involved if I wanted that information, at a cost of several hundred dollars.

The question arises as to how the FDA could declare Entelev/CanCell ineffective. According to NCI testing results (printed beginning on page 60), they conducted two official In-Vitro tests: Experiment ID: 9011NS78, Test Date November 19, 1990 and Experiment ID: 9102RG51, Test Date February 5, 1991. Both reports clearly show that CanCell was effective against all of the fifty-eight different strains of human cancer tested. In every case, the Percentage Growth lists the results in negative numbers, indicating reduction in the size of every tumor. For instance, a -50 indicates that the tumor was reduced by one-half; a -100 that the tumor was eliminated entirely. Since the testing time was short of that specified by Sheridan, it may be assumed that if it had been done in the correct time frame the results would have been even more spectacular.

It is obvious that this entire matter deserves a fair and just hearing by an impartial body to separate fact from fiction. The CanCell/Entelev hypothesis represents a new theory about the cause and cure of cancer. The old theories that have been the basis for all research for the past fifty years have brought no sure cure for cancer except surgery in limited specific cases.

Mr. Sopcak has reproduced in a handout the following quotations, which serve to soothe the insulted common sense of many people who have observed first-hand the effects of cancer treatment:

> Hardin Jones, of the University of California, Berkeley, stated: "For a typical cancer, people who refused treatment live an average of 12.5 years. Those who accept surgery and other kinds of treatment lived an average of only three years."

> And Dr. Lana Levi, of the University of California, wrote, in 1987, that: "Most cancer patients in this country die of chemotherapy. . .It does not eliminate breast, colon or lung cancer. This fact has been known for over a decade. . .Women with breast cancer are likely to die faster with chemotherapy than without it."

DEPARTMENT OF HEALTH & HUMAN SERVICES   Public Health Service

National Institutes of Health
National Cancer Institute
Bethesda, Maryland 20892

October 2, 1990

Mr. James V. Sheridan
17750 Castle
Roseville, Michigan 48066

Dear Mr. Sheridan:

Over ten years ago, the National Cancer Institute screened a preparation of yours, JS-101, in our in vivo anticancer screen. The compound was determined to be inactive. Recently, a major restructuring of the NCI's anticancer drug screening program was completed, and we have begun to screen selected compounds in this new system. This initiative represents a shift in emphasis from a "compound-oriented" strategy to a specific "disease-oriented" approach, focusing on major solid tumor types. In making this change, the former high-capacity in vivo prescreen model, the mouse leukemia P388, has been replaced by a new in vitro system consisting of panels of human tumor cell lines. Presently, the cell line panel consists of 60 lines, organized into seven subpanels including leukemia, lung, colon, renal, ovary, melanoma, and brain cancers. A recent article outlining this new program is enclosed for your reference.

We would be interested in evaluating your material referred to as Entelev, Cancel or JS-101 in our new in vitro test system provided you are able to supply us with additional material. In general, 10-25 mg samples of materials supplied in solid form are required for the initial assay. If, however, the sample is supplied as a solution, we will require approximately 50 mls in order to test the compound at full strength.

Please feel free to contact us if you have any questions. We look forward to receiving the sample.

Sincerely yours,

Ven L. Narayanan, Ph.D.
Chief, Drug Synthesis & Chemistry Branch
National Cancer Institute
Executive Plaza North, Room 831
Bethesda, MD 20892

VLN:lm

cc: Dr. Chabner
    Dolores Daly

Enclosure

17550 Castle
Roseville, Mi. 48066

October 15, 1990

Ven L. Narayanan, Ph. D.
Chief, Drug Synthesis & Chemistry Branch
National Cancer Institute
Executive Plaza North, Room 831
Bethesda, Md. 20892

Dear Dr. Narayanan:

Thank you for your letter dated October 2, 1990 and your offer to test Entelev/Cancell in your new testing method.

Attached is a pint sample of the material. The concentration is 200 mg./ml. There does not appear to be any toxicity to normal cells.

A sheet of graphs is enclosed. The "lytic activity" test seems to be similar to the new test you describe.

For the record, may I correct a misstatement in your letter. You say your testsof over ten years ago "determined the compound to be inactive". This statement is incorrect.

In your test you did something wrong. I called it to your attention.

You repeated the test Five (5) additional times. Despite my repeated letters and phone calls you repeated the error all five (5) times. Running the test incorrectly six (6) times does not justify your conclusion.

Sincerely yours,

James V. Sheridan

JVS/eas
Enclosure

DEPARTMENT OF HEALTH & HUMAN SERVICES

Public Health Service

National Institutes of Heal
National Cancer Institute
Bethesda, Maryland 208!
Telex: 908111

December 21, 1990

Mr. James V. Sheridan
17550 Castle
Roseville, MI 48066

Dear Mr. Sheridan,

The NCI's new investigational *in vitro* disease-oriented primary antitumor screen has now entered a fully operational phase. A recent description of the rationale, background, current status and other details are provided in the enclosed review from PPO Updates. Currently, the cell panel consists of 60 lines against which compounds are tested at a minimum of five concentrations at 10-fold dilutions. A 48 hour continuous drug exposure protocol is used, and a sulforhodamine B (SRB) protein assay is used to estimate cell viability or growth.

The development and applications of numerical and statistical methods of screening data analysis and refinement of selection criteria is continuing. However, we have adopted, on an interim basis, a set of data display and analysis procedures described briefly in the attachments provided. Pilot studies performed during the past 1 1/2 years have provided the basis for calibration of the screen with respect to known standards and the development of methods to facilitate the detection of patterns of interest.

The checklist includes observations of the mean response parameters, differential cellular sensitivity, and any subpanel-specific patterns of sensitivity. Enclosed are data obtained in the current operational screening protocol on compound(s) submitted by you recently and/or during the earlier development or pilot phases of the new *in vitro* screen. Screening program staff have reviewed the data and have provided the attached summary checklist for your information. Also indicated is any further pending action by NCI.

Our staff welcomes your comments, criticisms, and advice concerning the information provided and the display formats employed. If you have specific questions concerning the enclosed data, or the status of your compounds, please contact Dr. K. Paull, Chief, Information Technology Branch (Fax 301-496-8333) or Dr. Ven Narayanan, Chief, Drug Synthesis and Chemistry Branch (Phone 301-496-8795, Fax 301-496-8333).

Michael R. Boyd   MD PhD

NCI Developmental Therapeutics Program Dose Response Matrix	NSC: 637907-L/ 1	Exp. ID: 9011NS78
	Test Date: November 19, 1990	Stain: PRO
	Report Date: December 23, 1990	SSPL:

Log₁₀ Concentration (ug/ml)	Panel/Cell Line	Log₁₀ GI50	GI50

PG (0.9) 4.9 3.9 2.9 1.9 0.9	Panel/Cell Line	Log₁₀ GI50	GI50
13	• Leukemia CCRF-CEM	< 0.90	
15	HL-60(TB)	< 0.90	
77	K-562	1.21	
31	MOLT-4	< 0.90	
61	RPMI-8226	1.04	
34	SR	< 0.90	
55	Non-Small Cell Lung Cancer A549/ATCC	0.96	
99	HOP-18	2.06	
84	HOP-62	1.40	
91	HOP-92	1.29	
97	NCI-H226	1.29	
73	NCI-H322M	1.04	
48	NCI-H460	< 0.90	
31	NCI-H522	< 0.90	
73	LXFL-529L	1.04	
22	• Small Cell Lung Cancer DMS 114	< 0.90	
60	DMS 273	0.98	
88	Colon Cancer COLO 205	1.11	
77	DLD-1	1.14	
82	HCC-2998	1.34	
71	HCT-116	1.03	
65	HCT-15	1.00	
85	HT29	1.17	
67	KM12	1.06	
86	KM20L2	1.15	
77	SW-620	1.07	
61	CNS Cancer SF-268	0.98	
95	SF-295	1.14	
77	SF-539	1.26	
86	SNB-19	1.93	
95	SNB-75	1.26	
80	SNB-78	1.17	
72	U251	1.03	
60	Melanoma LOX IMVI	0.96	
75	MALME-3M	1.49	
79	M14	1.06	
62	M19-MEL	0.99	
93	SK-MEL-2	1.50	
90	SK-MEL-28	1.20	
67	SK-MEL-5	1.01	
83	UACC-257	1.09	
121	UACC-62	1.07	
84	Ovarian Cancer IGROV1	1.62	
68	OVCAR-3	1.01	
77	OVCAR-4	1.06	
92	OVCAR-5	1.12	
72	OVCAR-8	1.05	
96	SK-OV-3	1.36	
66	Renal Cancer 786-0	1.00	
93	A498	1.93	
65	ACHN	1.09	
92	CAKI-1	1.89	
81	RXF-393	1.08	
34	RXF-631	< 0.90	
74	SN12C	1.05	
103	TK-10	1.76	
90	UO-31	1.94	

+4 +3 +2 +1 0 -1 -2 -3

	PG > GI50	D₍GI50₎ = 58.8 (0.9)	MG MID GI50 = 1.19
	PG ≤ GI50	D₍TGI₎ = 24.5 (1.9)	Delta = 0.28
	PG ≤ TGI	D₍LC50₎ = 54.5 (1.9)	Range = 1.16
	PG ≤ LC50	D₍H₎ = 81.12 (0.9)	MGD₍H₎ = 75.45

NUMERICAL CHART OF NUMBERS DEPICTED ON GRAPH

NATIONAL CANCER INSTITUTE DEVELOPMENTAL THERAPEUTICS PROGRAM

In-Vitro Testing Results NSC: 637907-L/ 1

Experiment ID: 9011N578   Test Type: 8   Report Date: Dec. 23, 1990   Test Date: Nov. 13,1990

Stain Reagent:PRO

CELL LINE	Concentration of Cancer (Percentage Growth) Units: ug/ml Log 10				
	0.9	1.9	2.9	3.9	log 10 µg/ml)
	(10)	(100)	(1,000)	(10,000)	µg/ml approximate concentration
LEUKEMIA					
CCRF-CEM	13.7	-1.6	-0.5	-2.9	
HL-60(TB)	14.7	-28.3	-62.6	-19.4	
K-562	77.4	-12.1	0.0	3.3	
MOLT-4	31.2	-12.4	0.6	0.0	
RPMI-8226	61.5	-21.1	2.4	-8.1	
SR	34.0	-27.6	-24.7	-33.0	
NON-SMALL CELL LUNG CANCER					
A549/ATCC	55.4	-49.1	-26.7	-19.0	
HOP-18	99.0	68.4	-44.6	-36.9	
HOP-62	83.9	15.9	-80.2	-42.5	
HOP-92	91.2	-16.2	-51.9	-31.2	
NCI-H226	97.4	-23.5	-51.3	-34.1	

NCI-H23   The chart provided Mr. Sheridan by NCI did not include any numbers for Percentage Growth for this cell line of NonSmall Cell Lung Cancer.

NCI-H322M	73.5	-100.0	-48.3	-22.2	
NCI-H460	47.9	-72.4	-60.2	-14.6	
NCI-H522	30.5	-86.1	-38.7	-17.7	
LXFL-529	73.0	-95.5	-60.5	-15.3	
SMALL CELL LUNG CANCER					
DMS 114	21.6	-86.2	-74.1	-32.4	
DMS 273	59.9	-67.9	-43.2	-14.9	
COLON CANCER					
COLO 205	87.8	-97.6	-93.4	-51.2	
DLD-1	76.9	-38.1	-22.6	-9.6	
HCC-2998	82.2	8.7	-68.3	-38.4	
HCT-116	70.9	-99.2	-95.8	-63.5	
HCT-15	65.0	-89.0	-66.7	-37.3	
HT29	84.6	-44.5	-58.7	-29.1	
KM12	67.2	-44.4	-88.8	-6.9	
KM20L2	86.4	-64.0	-70.1	-36.3	
SW-620	76.7	-79.6	-24.2	-37.1	
CNS CANCER					
SF-268	60.6	-83.5	-38.1	-14.7	
SF-295	94.8	-94.6	-54.8	-18.6	
SF-539	77.2	1.1	-56.2	-7.9	
SNB-19	86.1	53.9	-90.3	-38.2	
SNB-75	95.2	-32.6	-80.4	-33.2	
SNB-78	80.1	-32.6	-33.1	-36.8	
U251	71.6	-98.8	-77.2	-14.4	

CELL LINE	Concentration of Cancer (Percentage Growth) Units: ug/ml Log 10			
	0.9	1.9	2.9	3.9 log 10 µg/ml)
	(10)	(100)	(1,000)	(10,000) µg/ml approximate concentration
MELANOMA				
LOX IMVI	59.5	-98.0	-96.9	-70.0
MALME-3M	74.9	32.8	-58.1	-31.8
MI4	78.6	-98.0	-76.3	-10.8
MI9-MEL-	62.2	-85.6	-71.6	-29.0
SK-MEL-2	93.0	21.0	-33.2	-10.3
SK-MEL-28	89.9	-42.2	-50.3	-11.5.
SK-MEL-5	67.3	-95.8	-88.4	-38.8
UACC-257	83.3	-91.4	-77.9	-47.7
UACC-62	79.7	-98.9	-88.1	-28.3
OVARIAN CANCER				
IGROVI	83.8	36.7-	-40.8	-24.6
OVCAR-3	67.6	-99.8	-62.0	-22.8
OVCAR-4	77.5	-94.7	-35.9	-11.6
OVCAR-5	92.3	-99.6	-99.3	-64.7
OVCAR-8	72.1	-82.2	-60.0	0.4
SK-OV-3	95.5	-4.0	-46.4	-29.9
RENAL CANCER				
786-0	66.3	-100.0	-81.3	-7.3
A498	93.2	54.2	-85.7	-65.2
ACHN	65.1	-17.4	-81.6	-11.3
CAKI-I	92.0	49.2	-22.2	-17.6
RXF-393	80.5	-96.5	-97.6	-56.0
RXF-631	34.0	-21.6	-25.3	-29.4
SN12C	74.3	-98.0	-61.9	-10.5
TK-10	102.9	41.0	-51.9	-100.0
UO-31	90.0	54.6	-89.6	-29.2

National Cancer Institute Developmental Therapeutics Program
In-Vitro Screening Data Review Checklist

C: 637907-L/ 1	Experiment ID: 9011NS78	Source:
st Date: November 19, 1990	Review Date: 1/11/9 1	

Review Summary

1. MG_MID Response Parameters

   a. Log_{10} GI50   1.19
   b. Log_{10} TGI   1.62
   c. Log_{10} LC50   3.25

2. Selectivity Analysis

   a. Differential Cellular Sensitivity

       (1) GI50   0.28
       (2) TGI   0.51
       (3) LC50   1.65

   (Low |delta<1|=L., Mod |1<delta<3|=M, High|delta>=3|=H)

   b. Differential Subpanel Sensitivity

   Subpanels* showing a statistical measure of differential sensitivity (see definition and derivation attached) with respect to the indicated response parameter (GI50, TGI, or LC50)

	Response Parameter	Subpanel Specificity		
(1)	GI50	LEU		
(2)	TGI	LEU	SCL	
(3)	LC50	SCL		

   * Tumor cell line subpanels are identified as follows:
CNS = Brain;	COL = Colon;	LEU = Leukemia/Lymphoma;
LNS = Non-small Cell Lung;	MEL = Melanoma;	MIS = Miscellaneous
OVA = Ovary;	REN = Kidney;	SCL = Small Cell Lung;

Pending Action by NCI

1. _____ None
2. ___✓___ Repeat testing in Primary Screen
        5 Log_{10} _____ ;   10 Log_{10} _____ ;   Other _____.
3. _____ Refer to Biological Evaluation Committee
4. _____ Refer to Natural Products Program Committee

National Cancer Institute Developmental Therapeutics Program
In-Vitro Testing Results

NSC: 637907 -L/1	Experiment ID: 9102RG51	Test Type: 8	Units: ug/ml
Report Date: August 26, 1992	Test Date: February 5, 1991	QNS:	MC:
COMI: Cancell	Stain Reagent: PROTEIN-51	SSPL: F71A	

Panel/Cell Line	Time Zero	Ctrl	Mean Optical Densities -0.1	0.9	1.9	2.9	3.9	Percent Growth -0.1	0.9	1.9	2.9	3.9	GI50	TGI	LC50
Leukemia															
CCRF-CEM	0.376	1.532	1.150	0.552	0.279	0.280	0.193	67	15	-26	-26	-49	1.70E+00	1.88E+01	>8.00E+03
HL-60 (TB)	0.611	2.190	2.076	0.492	0.398	0.241	0.145	93	-20	-35	-61	-76	1.92E+00	5.36E+00	3.10E+02
K-562	0.217	1.486	1.526	1.132	0.126	0.146	0.142	103	72	-42	-33	-34	1.25E+01	3.43E+01	>8.00E+03
MOLT-4	0.649	2.187	2.000	1.060	0.457	0.333	0.234	88	27	-30	-49	-64	3.33E+00	2.39E+01	9.65E+02
RPMI-8226	0.643	2.139	1.785	1.236	0.453	0.356	0.292	76	40	-30	-45	-55	4.19E+00	2.99E+01	2.74E+03
SR	.	.	.	.	.	.	.	.	.	.	.	.	.	.	.
Non-Small Cell Lung Cancer															
A549/ATCC	0.489	2.156	2.202	1.358	0.491	0.367	0.354	103	52	0	-25	-28	8.77E+00	8.07E+01	>8.00E+03
EKVX	0.747	1.384	1.386	1.322	0.741	0.511	0.475	100	90	-1	-32	-36	2.21E+01	7.83E+01	>6.00E+03
HOP-18	0.862	.	1.015	0.928	0.873	0.082	0.530	.	.	.	.	.	.	.	.
HOP-62	1.261	1.902	1.943	1.863	1.248	0.040	0.620	107	94	-3	-97	-52	2.27E+01	7.52E+01	2.55E+02
HOP-92	0.936	1.372	1.378	1.285	0.858	0.442	0.543	101	80	-8	-53	-42	1.75E+01	6.44E+01	.
NCI-H23	0.564	1.420	1.403	1.213	0.287	0.330	0.286	98	76	-49	-41	-49	1.29E+01	3.24E+01	>8.00E+03
NCI-H322M	0.447	1.033	1.069	0.972	0.045	0.194	0.193	106	90	-90	-56	-57	1.33E+01	2.52E+01	4.79E+01
NCI-H460	0.273	1.826	1.780	1.082	0.115	0.144	0.170	97	52	-58	-47	-38	8.36E+00	2.38E+01	.
NCI-H522	0.626	1.126	0.699	0.585	0.173	0.371	0.301	55	-7	-72	-41	-52	9.53E-01	6.24E+00	.
LXFL 529	0.493	1.887	1.871	1.480	0.024	0.158	0.270	99	71	-95	-68	-45	1.07E+01	2.14E+01	.
Small Cell Lung Cancer															
DMS 114	0.649	1.711	1.574	0.933	0.469	0.275	0.362	87	27	-28	-58	-44	3.29E+00	2.48E+01	.
DMS 273	0.226	1.056	1.042	0.611	0.104	0.139	0.137	98	46	-54	-38	-39	6.81E+00	2.31E+01	.
Colon Cancer															
COLO 205	0.443	1.657	1.766	1.623	0.093	0.085	0.098	111	97	-79	-81	-78	1.48E+01	2.85E+01	5.47E+01
DLD-1	0.462	1.606	1.643	1.331	0.392	0.243	0.180	103	76	-15	-48	-61	1.54E+01	5.44E+01	1.22E+01
HCC-2998	0.891	1.812	1.955	1.462	0.454	0.166	0.229	115	62	-49	-81	-74	1.02E+01	2.89E+01	6.53E+01
HCT-116	0.253	1.653	1.615	1.260	0.015	0.023	0.082	97	72	-94	-91	-68	1.06E+01	2.17E+01	4.33E+01
HCT-15	0.443	1.659	1.616	1.152	0.436	0.280	0.282	97	56	-1	-37	-36	1.10E+01	7.69E+01	>8.00E+03
HT29	0.243	1.319	1.410	1.159	0.201	0.212	0.130	108	85	-17	-13	-47	1.76E+01	5.42E+01	>8.00E+03
KM12	0.316	1.507	1.276	0.969	0.046	0.102	0.172	61	55	-65	-68	-46	8.66E+00	1.97E+01	.
KM20L2	0.488	1.897	2.043	1.367	0.267	0.338	0.256	110	64	-45	-31	-48	1.07E+01	3.07E+01	>8.00E+03
SW-620	0.319	1.692	1.572	1.216	0.131	0.196	0.139	91	65	-59	-39	-57	1.06E+01	2.68E+01	.
CNS Cancer															
SF-268	0.53e	1.640	1.541	1.161	0.139	0.240	0.285	91	56	-74	-55	-47	9.25E+00	2.21E+01	.
SF-295	0.564	1.463	1.479	1.436	0.054	0.160	0.346	102	97	-91	-72	-39	1.43E+01	2.64E+01	.
SF-539	0.609	1.421	1.518	1.270	0.606	0.107	0.287	112	82	0	-63	-53	1.94E+01	7.89E+01	3.21E+02
SNB-19	0.570	1.444	1.456	1.313	0.846	0.030	0.300	101	85	32	-95	.	3.62E+01	1.42E+02	3.54E+02
SNB-75	0.496	0.625	0.612	0.780	0.561	0.077	0.280	96	86	26	-84	-43	3.18E+01	1.37E+02	.
SNB-78	0.731	1.385	1.410	1.363	0.737	0.533	0.469	104	97	1	-27	-36	2.46E+01	6.63E+01	>6.00E+03
U251	0.519	1.782	1.911	1.526	0.405	0.280	0.296	110	80	-22	-46	-43	1.57E+01	4.67E+01	>8.00E+03
XF 498	0.902	1.256	1.262	1.148	0.174	0.526	0.502	102	69	-81	-42	-44	1.08E+01	2.32E+01	.
Melanoma															
LOX IMVI	0.250	1.403	1.285	0.935	0.079	0.052	0.135	90	59	-68	-79	-46	9.48E+00	2.33E+01	.
MALME-3M	0.727	1.931	1.910	1.842	1.490	0.339	0.544	96	93	63	-53	-25	1.04E+02	2.79E+02	.
M14	0.377	1.462	1.529	1.356	0.135	0.064	0.134	106	90	-64	-83	-64	1.46E+01	3.07E+01	6.47E+01
M19-MEL	0.318	1.122	1.172	0.841	0.042	0.144	0.179	106	65	-87	-55	-44	1.01E+01	2.15E+01	.
SK-MEL-2	0.604	1.372	1.456	1.271	1.003	0.292	0.301	111	87	52	-52	-50	8.36E+01	2.54E+02	7.73E+02
SK-MEL-28	0.402	1.119	1.076	0.973	0.524	0.151	0.197	94	80	17	-63	-51	2.37E+01	1.31E+02	5.56E+02
SK-MEL-5	0.620	.	2.071	1.685	0.528	0.183	0.197	.	.	.	.	.	.	.	.
UACC-257	0.597	1.366	1.423	1.299	0.677	0.448	0.330	107	91	10	-25	-45	2.59E+01	1.57E+02	>6.00E+03
UACC-62	0.717	1.970	2.026	1.863	0.538	0.286	0.382	104	91	-25	-60	-47	1.82E+01	4.88E+01	.
Ovarian Cancer															
IGROV1	0.655	1.793	1.953	1.725	0.954	0.208	0.386	114	94	26	-68	-41	3.57E+01	1.52E+02	.
OVCAR-3	0.564	1.174	1.105	0.809	0.167	0.430	0.319	89	40	-70	-24	-43	4.99E+00	1.84E+01	.
OVCAR-4	0.741	1.426	1.385	1.227	0.005	0.007	0.401	94	71	-99	-99	-46	1.06E+01	2.09E+01	.
OVCAR-5	0.641	1.645	1.587	1.687	0.089	0.220	0.426	94	104	-86	-66	-34	1.54E+01	2.82E+01	.
OVCAR-8	0.402	1.386	1.408	1.196	0.241	0.280	0.268	102	81	-40	-30	-33	1.44E+01	3.73E+01	>8.00E+03
SK-OV-3	0.746	0.987	1.032	1.045	0.907	0.211	0.383	119	124	67	-72	-49	1.06E+02	2.43E+02	.
Renal Cancer															
766-0	0.265	1.466	1.531	1.191	-0.009	0.013	0.139	105	77	-100	-95	-48	1.14E+01	2.16E+01	.
A498	1.091	1.488	1.451	1.398	1.170	0.036	0.013	91	77	20	-97	.	2.40E+01	1.19E+02	3.19E+02
ACHN	0.464	1.475	1.423	1.164	0.206	0.275	0.315	95	69	-56	-41	-32	1.14E+01	2.66E+01	.
CAKI-1	0.514	1.860	1.796	1.306	0.029	0.268	0.340	95	59	-94	-48	-34	9.13E+00	1.94E+01	.
RXF-631	0.456	1.149	1.168	1.033	0.105	0.173	0.303	103	83	-77	-62	-34	1.29E+01	2.65E+01	.
SN12C	0.716	1.732	1.729	1.327	0.029	0.047	0.430	100	60	-96	-93	-40	9.28E+00	1.94E+01	.
TK-10	0.830	1.417	1.401	1.376	0.916	0.588	0.517	97	93	15	-29	-38	2.84E+01	1.73E+02	>8.00E+03
UO-31	0.680	1.136	1.065	0.956	0.794	0.440	0.373	84	61	25	-35	-45	1.60E+01	2.08E+02	>8.00E+03

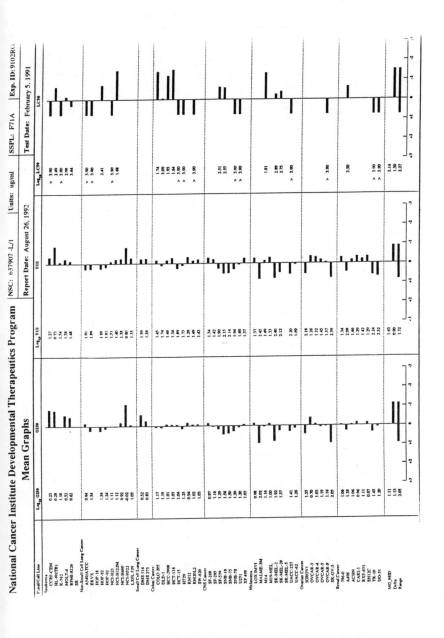

National Cancer Institute Developmental Therapeutics Program

Mean Graphs

NSC: 637907 -L/1 | Units: ug/ml

Report Date: August 26, 1992

Exp. ID: 9102RG

SSPL: F71A | Test Date: February 5, 1991

National Cancer Institute Developmental Therapeutics Program
Dose Response Curves

NSC: 637907 -L/1	SSPL: F71A	Exp. ID: 9102RG51
Report Date: August 26, 1992	Test Date: February 5, 1991	

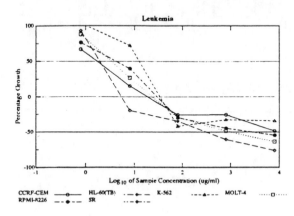

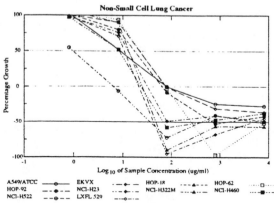

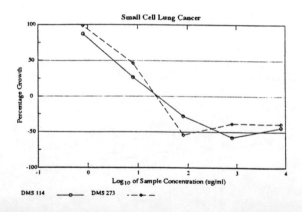

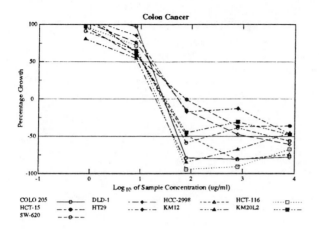

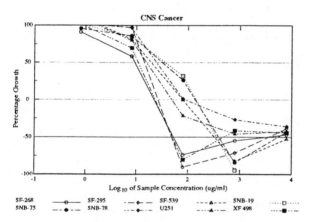

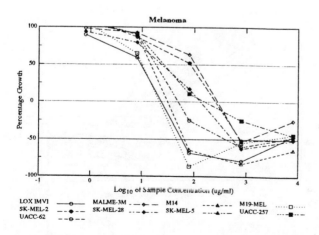

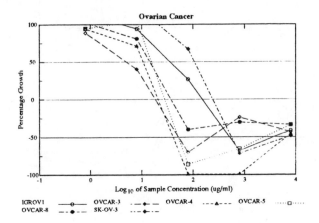

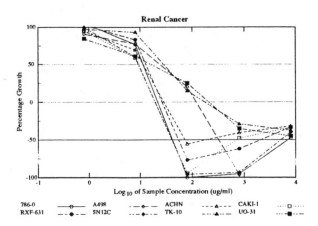

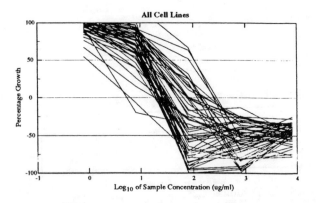

Controversy about the NCI In-Vitro test results, along with the letters and Sheridan's accounts of faulty procedures, indicate that people in charge there lack understanding of their own programs. Test data discrepancies further suggest undisciplined lack of attention to details.

A simple explanation is in order. In-Vitro testing refers to work done using cancer specimens grown in a laboratory, as opposed to clinical testing, which refers to work done using patients. Confusion arises when people who are not conversant with charts and who do not know how to interpret them make incorrect assumptions. When a minus sign (-) is placed before a number reporting tumor growth, it represents a percent reduction in the size of the tumor. A plus sign (+) indicates increased growth. A -100 would indicate that all of the tumor was eliminated; a +50 would indicate that the tumor had increased by 50 percent.

Some executives at the American Cancer Society, along with "quack busters" hired by various pharmaceutical companies, reported the minus signs indicated CanCell failures. In fact, because cancers in various locations need different time allowances to be eradicated by CanCell, Sopcak maintains that if correct protocol had been followed, all the cancers would have been completely eliminated and all would have had -100 growth. If CanCell were not effective, the tumors would have grown and the percentage of growth would have been noted with a plus sign (+) before each number. There was not a single plus sign reported.

4
The History of Entelev and CanCell

James V. Sheridan, the inspired chemist who invented Entelev. Edward J. Sopcak, the metallurgist who succeeded him and developed CanCell. The present status of the materials.

James V. Sheridan remembers September 6, 1936, as the date he started his Entelev project. Years later, beginning in the 1940s, he finally had perfected the formula and began distributing it free of charge to any cancer patient who asked for it. He believed that his inexpensive cure would ultimately be recognized by the medical community and he would make it available to anyone for the price of manufacture and delivery. A man deeply committed to the service of humanity, he vowed that he would never use the formula to make a profit.

He engaged in a series of efforts, following established rules of procedure, that moved him from one workplace to another in an effort to bring his formula to the attention of cancer research organizations. He was determined to have Entelev professionally tested, its value recognized, and the material ultimately approved by the Food and Drug Administration.

While he worked through professional channels to achieve his goal, he continued to produce and give the material to cancer patients. In his personal effort to save lives, he was in fact conducting a kind of grass-roots testing program, although today he has precious little scientifically prepared documentation of the fact. He had neither the sophisticated training nor the financial wherewithal to keep the kind of quality records demanded by today's established medical service industry. He does claim to have lists of patients and their letters of personal success with Entelev, however.

The real proof of the efficacy of Entelev can be estimated only by the fact that he passed out thousands of free bottles of the material as a result of its success being spread by word of mouth from patient to patient. Such generous recognition of a product's value comes easily to the terminal cancer patient, whose only interest is in results; but it is almost impossible to elicit from the medical service industry representatives, who demand to know the how and why of those results. The medical service industry itself, however, provides precious little follow-up statistics about its own success or failure rate after their formulas leave the labs. They require no more follow-up record-keeping of patients than Sheridan did. Business reserves its best monitoring for its financial reporting.

After years of working through established channels with dogged determination, and being plagued by a series of questionable circumstances, Sheridan decided to quit the project in 1983. He was convinced that a conspiracy existed, prompted by the medical services industry and abetted by people in charge of the American Cancer Society, the NCI and the FDA, to prevent the finding of a cure for cancer in order to protect private financial interests. He concluded that his battle was not now with cancer, for he had won that. His battle now was with the forces of greed, and it was a political battle for which he was not prepared. Tired and dejected, he simply walked away from the project that had dominated his life.

About that time, there was a terminal cancer patient, Don Wilson, lying in St. Joseph Hospital in Ann Arbor, Michigan. He had been given the traditional chemotherapy treatment for cancer and suffered the traditional side effects, including kidney damage which ultimately caused the renal failure that cost him his life. While he was lying there waiting to die, he decided to try Entelev in a last-ditch effort to cure his cancer. After using Entelev for a period of six weeks, he left the hospital free of cancer.

Mr. Wilson decided he wanted to keep using Entelev as a kind of security blanket, but he soon discovered that it was no longer available because Sheridan had stopped making it. He talked about this dilemma with a friend, Orville Feather. Mr. Feather, in turn, discussed the situation with his friend, Edward J. Sopcak, who volunteered to make Entelev for Wilson if he could get the formula. Sheridan freely provided it, grateful to have someone willing and able to carry on his work.

Soon Sopcak had taken up where Sheridan left off, manufacturing the product in his home and distributing it free of charge to any cancer patient who requested it. When Sopcak started making and distributing the formula, he changed the name of the product to CanCell in order to avoid infringement on Sheridan's name, Entelev. He also began to modify and change the formula.

After a while, Sopcak attracted a following of volunteers who organized to help in his efforts and a rather primitive system of record-keeping was established. Sopcak had been passing out his own private telephone number and talking to patients every evening, listening to their cancer stories and filling their requests for CanCell. Now volunteers established a headquarters in Milford, Michigan, and started manning telephones using a CanCell Request Line phone number, 1-313-684-5529. A protocol for requests was determined and patients were required to fill out re-order forms that included a simple progress report.

Today Sopcak estimates that he has given out over 30,000 bottles of treatments and has received over 5,000 letters of appreciation testifying to the success of CanCell. He admits to being so busy making and distributing the product that he devoted little time or money to record-keeping. Since the FDA filed a petition in federal court that resulted in an injunction ordering him to stop making and distributing CanCell in November of 1992, volunteers have been engaged in a concentrated effort to computerize records and complete a mailing list to identify participants. If lax record-keeping seems strange in today's world, remember that the production and distribution of CanCell, just as that of Entelev before it, was done after working hours, as a humanitarian effort. Mr. Sopcak runs a business by day to earn a living and support his efforts on behalf of CanCell. He used his limited time and financial resources on results-oriented production and distribution.

In attempting to estimate the number of people who have successfully used CanCell, a skeptical Sopcak speculates that a rather large number of requests he filled may have gone to people who were laying by a supply for future use in case they ever became cancer victims.

In June 1990, a disappointed Sheridan wrote a heartfelt accounting of his experiences, which he circulated free of charge to anyone to read, copy and pass along to others. He tells his own story in a simple unsophisticated style, reflecting an unfaltering belief in his findings and a sense of hope that remains intact despite all of his reversals. A re-typed copy is printed here, Document No. 6.:

The History of Entelev/CanCell
by Jim Sheridan

I have been asked to tell a little about my background and then to tell the story behind the material—first called Entelev and later called CanCell.

I was born in 1912, in Northeastern Pennsylvania, in the town of Ireskow (a mining town). Nearby was the town of Coleraine (a mining town), where my dad was born and raised. My father and both grandfathers were coal miners. I failed to escape completely the coal mining gene and worked 4 months in a coal strip mine.

In the middle of all these coal fields was the city of Hazelton, where I was raised from a little tad to a high school graduate. What I remember most about those years is that I completed 2 years of Junior High in one year; that during 2 years of high school I worked 15 hours per week in a clothing store; and that during the other 2 years it was 54 hours per week running an elevator. I graduated from high school in 1929. In the meantime, I had a State Senatorial Scholarship which pretty well covered tuition at the college of my choice.

The college of my choice was Carnegie Tech. I had decided I wanted to be a mining engineer and Carnegie Tech was said to have the best mining engineering course in the country. However, somewhere in my freshman year all thoughts of mining and engineering of any kind disappeared from my mind. It became very apparent that I was destined to be a chemist.

I spent 5 years at Carnegie Tech—4 years as an undergraduate, and 1 year as a graduate student. During my graduate year, I was a member of the teaching staff. (I could not have survived on a fellowship.) In addition, I had attended one summer school at Tech and one at the University of Pittsburgh. By the time I finished Tech, I had taken every advanced course in chemistry, physics, and math taught there. Meanwhile, meals were being earned by waiting on tables and washing dishes.

I went to Dow Chemical Co. in 1935, to work in the analytical lab. I was shifted to the Patent Dept. in 1937 and became a registered patent agent several years later.

In the meantime, the rules of practicing law were changed and one was required to pass the State Bar Exam and become a registered attorney at law in order to practice. Dow formed a law class, provided an instructor and, after about 5 years of home study, I passed the Michigan Bar Exam. I left Dow in 1946, went to Detroit, and earned a living doing patent work until 1950.

Now back to 1931, to chemistry, and to the research project. There were two events in 1931, and a dream in 1936, which mark the beginning of the project. On a Friday evening in April of 1931 (in my sophomore year at Tech,) I was working in an analytical chemistry lab. That evening the school was having an "open house" for the benefit of high school students and their parents. We students were to do that evening what we normally would have done that Friday afternoon. I was at a step in the analysis which resulted in a beaker full of a yellow colored liquid. Normally, this liquid would have been discarded but, in this case, it was still sitting there on the lab bench. Two high school boys came by and one of these asked, "Is that color due to chromate?"

I said, "Yes."

He said, "How would you change that color?"

I said, "Just add an acid. It will produce a bright red color."

He said, "What acid?"

I said, "Any acid—here, I will show you."

I went to a shelf of acids and picked one at random. I added it to the yellow liquid and got the surprise of my life. The liquid broke into 6 bands of color—the rainbow colors in rainbow order. Red-orange-yellow-green-blue-violet.

The boy's eyes popped out and my eyes double-popped out. The entire class and several professors gathered around. Others in the class, who had their "yellow solution," tried it and it worked. However, no other acid worked.

One of the professors said, "That looks like a case of 'rhythmic banding' and, if it is, the width of each band will be 2.7 times the width of the band above it."

Sure enough, we measured the bands and, as near as we could measure it, each band was 2.7 times wider than the band above it.

So it was "rhythmic banding," whatever that means.

About a month after the "rhythmic banding," I was required to name the chemistry professor under whom I would do a research program during my Junior and Senior years. I picked Dr. John Warner, who was "Jake" to everyone. He later became President of Carnegie Tech and was still "Jake" to everyone. Jake had become interested in the Debye Theory which had been published in 1927. My task was to check out the validity of the theory by determining the effect of changes in dielectric constant on reactions between positive and negative ions.

This I did during my Junior, Senior and graduate years.

I started on my research assignment and my first big surprise was that Jake made me take a course he taught in graduate school—"Theory and Thermodynamics of Solutions." This was a course that required 2 years of physical chemistry—of which I hadn't yet had day one. And then he made me repeat the course during my Senior year—and again during my graduate year. Needless to say, after taking the courses three times, and doing three years of research on the Debye Theory, I was not likely to forget it very soon.

The third event, a dream, occurred on the afternoon of September 6, 1936, when I was taking a nap.

The dream brought together the event of the rainbow in the beaker and the work on the Debye Theory.

In the 1936 dream, the layers of the rainbow represented the respiratory enzymes. Each color represented an enzyme at a specific redox level. The electrons from the Debye Theory represented the energy units in the respiration moving from glucose to oxygen from that respiratory system.

Somehow, the dream suggested the possibility of a controlled altering of the pathway of energy flow and energy production in the respiratory system to: (A) cause a cancer or (B) cure a cancer.

When I woke up I felt that I had received my MARCHING ORDERS. Three years later I bought my first mice and I was on my way in my basement lab.

The suggested cure was to make the cancer cell even more primitive—to the point where the cancer cell would lyse (similar to digest).

I started a basement lab and started to treat tumor-bearing mice. Dow showed no interest in the work. I left Dow in 1946 and moved to Detroit, with the hope of generating interest in the area's colleges and research organizations.

Treatment of patients began in the late 1940s.

About 1950, I was invited to join the staff of the

Detroit Institute of Cancer Research (now the Michigan Cancer foundation). I did the chemical work required on the project and the Institute experts did the animal tests.

After about 3 years at the Institute I was 41 years old and about to learn the facts of life.

In late 1953, the Institute Director concluded that the Material was ready for a clinical program. In accordance with the rules at the time, the Director formed a committee of himself, the Dean of Medicine at Wayne University, and 3 oncologists from area hospitals.

The committee spent several days at the Institute, interviewed the experts who were treating the mice, reviewed the mouse results and decided that the Material was ready for a clinical program.

Meanwhile, Mr. Grant Clark of New York City, and representing the American Tobacco Co., had been following the work for some time. He sent three experts from the University of Virginia. They, too, spent several days going over everything and also decided that the Material was ready for a clinical program.

Mr. Clark then reported that a check had been written for four hundred and fifty thousand dollars ($450,000) and would be sent as soon as certain formalities were completed. He also stated this would be followed by any number of millions required.

The next step was taken by the Director of the Institute who informed the American Cancer Society. The latter requested a meeting for the following Sunday morning in New York City. The Director and the Dean of the Wayne Medical School attended the meeting.

They returned and reported.

IS THE READER READY?

They reported that the AMERICAN CANCER SOCIETY did not approve of the test because I had not proved I owned the idea.

The program was immediately halted and several months later I was fired!

NOTE to the reader: It is now 37 years later. If you ever discover who owns this idea, will you let me know? I would like to get the American Cancer Society's approval for a clinical test.

The next step in learning the facts of life occurred at Battelle Institute in Columbus, Ohio. I spent 2 years there (1961-63).

Again, the work was repeated.

Battelle was the site for testing materials for the National Cancer Institute (NCI). Anyone could send in a material and it would be tested. At the time the "5 day test" was being used. Incidently, I could not pass the 5 day test at that time. In my case it took about 20-22 days before the tumors started to disappear.

My lab was next to, and just a wall away from, the NCI lab. The technicians who did my testing were the same people who did the NCI testing.

After 2 years of repeating all the work already done, the Chief of Battelle's Biochemical Division, who was also the head of the NCI testing lab, asked the federal NCI office for permission to test my Material in their lab; that is, test it "on the other side of the wall" from my lab. They were asked that a single test be run using my procedure (up to 20 days) instead of theirs (5 days) and make the results part of their records.

They refused. Several months later, I was fired!

The next giant step in learning the facts of life involved the FDA.

Question: Where was the FDA in all this?

On April 9, 1982, I submitted to the FDA my "Notice of Claimed Investigational Exemption for a New Drug (IND) under section 505 (1)."

On May 20, 1982, they issued me IND 20258. The language of the IND implied, at the least, that everything was in order for a clinical program.

Later I received a telephone call from the FDA, stating that the Material had been put on "clinical hold" because of lack of "preclinical data which would allow us to assess the potential risk of the Material."

Four years later (April 17, 1986) I received a letter which repeated the previous holding.

The major problem in all of this was that the so-called "minimum lethal dose" study had not been made. The reason for this had been the lack of funds (bordering on abject poverty).

Finally, in the fall of 1986, a kind soul offered the money and I thought I was ready to go ahead with the minimum dose studies.

I made arrangements with a laboratory which, I was assured by experts, was the best in the United States. A supply of the Material was shipped and 2 days later I received my regular six-month visit from the FDA.

I told them of the shipment. They visited the lab. The lab people called off the study.

A friend of mine knew a staff member at the lab. The reason the study was called off was "because they couldn't afford to get in trouble with the FDA." The offer of financial help was withdrawn.

However, that episode was only the beginning of the end. Shortly after that event the FDA started a "reign of terror."

The major steps were:

1. The incident just recited.
2. A nationally recognized expert had:
   a. Run mice tests involving four different tumors.
   b. Run tissue culture studies of the Material against cancer cells.
   c. Gathered together medical records of 40-50 human patients who had been treated with the Material. He had stated openly that "This is the best Material ever developed in the history of mankind." However, the FDA arrived and I received a call from the expert saying, "Jim, will you please not mention my name in connection with this Material anymore?"
3. An official of a drug company had done some favors for me and we had established a pleasant relationship. I was suddenly told our relationship and my presence were at an end and because the FDA had arrived and, in his own words, "scared the hell out of me."
4. Another laboratory had permitted me to use certain of their analytical instruments. The FDA arrived and—need I say more?

5. A number of people, including physicians, reported to me that they had called the FDA and asked:

Question: "What is holding up FDA approval?"

Answer: (by FDA) "Sheridan refuses to do the required tests."

6. Etc., etc. and etc.

AIDS

While all this was going on, a nationally known expert checked the material against the AIDS virus. He reported privately that this Material "dissolved off or disintegrated the collagen coating of the virus."

Since that time, I have been told about well over 100 AIDS patients being treated and cured. As yet, not one failure has been reported to me.

GENITAL HERPES

Genital Herpes has produced the most surprising result, a surprisingly rapid effect. So far 15 genital herpes cases have been reported to me by physicians with positive cures in every case in 3 to 6 days!

CONCLUSION

I don't have the resources to do battle with the United States Government, or with the American Cancer Society, or with the "frightened to death" medical profession. These are groups whose leadership has become saturated with mediocrity. Their slogan is, "please do not upset us with new ideas—things are now so nice and comfortable." So, they are winning by default. Maybe I should say they think they are winning.

When in the past people became sick and tired of some nice comfortable government or control group, there came a thing called a revolution. To make further revolution unnecessary, there came a thing called an election. The word "election" simply means, "Let's hear the voice of the People."

In this case the manipulation is very simple and very effective. They say, "Before we can consider your application, you must carry out test X. However, we are going to use our great power to stop you from carrying out test X and any other tests. In the meantime, we will issue an injunction which says: "THOU SHALT NOT!"

I can hardly wait to see what form the revolution takes in the present project. I will guess it will be in the form of a "PEOPLE INJUNCTION."

Yes, I see tempers starting to seethe—tempers of previously dying people who remember how close they came to death before they heard of the much prayed for cure—tempers of those who had refused to believe their beloved government would stoop to actively engage in deliberately scaring respectable competent scientists from contributing to the evaluation of a promising Material.

I submit that all that is needed now is a little spark, and an explosion will occur; and the People will issue an injunction to the FDA, the NCI etc.

I hope no one will mind if I enjoy the revolution.

James V. Sheridan

In support of Sheridan's allegations concerning his two year stint (1961-63) at Battelle Institute in Columbus, Ohio, a re-typed copy of a letter from R.S. Davidson, Chief of Biosciences Research, Battelle Columbus Laboratories, which Mr. Davidson certified on 7-28-90 to be a faithful reproduction of a letter that he sent to Mr. W.A. Allen, Secretary of the Else U. Pardee Foundation, is printed here. (See Document No. 7, page 84.)

This letter presents the clearest written explanation by an informed participant in the history of Entelev of why Sheridan's hypothesis was never accepted for testing by the cancer research organizations that were in positions to do so. They simply didn't understand it and reacted by condemning it. Jim Sheridan was born in 1912 and is still living in Michigan. It is imperative that a comprehensive investigation and testing of his hypothesis begin as soon as possible so that he may be included in the work before it is too late for him to participate.

Edward J. Sopcak has not written a personal history as Sheridan did. He says he doesn't have time for that, but he does talk about his background. He was born in 1920 in Gary, Indiana, and was educated in Gary public schools, graduating from Emerson High School there. He was graduated from Purdue University in 1942 with a B.S. in Metallurgical Engineering. He served in the U.S. Air Force in England during World War II, supervising the repairing of B-24 bombers. He entered service as a Second Lieutenant and left with the rank of Captain. Today he owns and operates the Michigan Metallurgical Products Co., Inc., in Howell, Michigan. The company makes precision castings in aluminum, bronze and copper. A perfectionist with an appetite for doing the so-called impossible, Sopcak if often called upon to make castings that no one else wants to attempt.

As of December 1992, both men remain dedicated to serving humanity without receiving any financial gain for their efforts. However, the Sheridan and Sopcak alliance is not now as close at it once was. Although the two men remain friends, and they agree that both Entelev and CanCell cure cancer, they disagree about how the products work. Simply stated, the chemist Sheridan believes that the chemical components of his formula cause the cancer cells to lyse and initiate the cure for cancer in a strictly chemical reaction. The metallurgist Sopcak believes that the chemical components cause a change in the energy and vibrational frequencies of the cells, causing them to lyse and initiate the cure for cancer. Sopcak has changed the original formula to conform to his energy hypothesis and believes this results in a more reliable product that will produce an even higher success rate. The new CanCell puts the vibrational frequency of oxygen into the cell structure. Sopcak also believes that a holistic approach to health is vital and lays down some rules for patients that govern diet and exclude the use of tobacco and a number of other substances.

In Detroit, Michigan, on February 21, 1989, the FDA filed a statutory injunction proceeding against their CanCell operations. Mr. Sheridan did not contest the complaint and on June 21, 1989, he consented to entry of a Decree of Permanent Injunction and quit his association with CanCell. The Government filed a motion for summary judgment against Sopcak's operation in December 1989, and on January 17, 1990, U.S. District Judge Bernard A. Friedman granted the motion. Sopcak continued to distribute CanCell, in violation of the Decree of Permanent Injunction, defending his actions as his constitutional right and humanitarian duty to save lives. On November 19, 1992, Judge Friedman found Sopcak in contempt of the Decree and ordered compliance. Sopcak stopped manufacture and distribution of CanCell and commenced preparing an appeal.

Sopcak graciously and freely credits Sheridan's original research and formulation of Entelev as the inspiration for his own involvement in cancer research that resulted in the development of CanCell. Sheridan's family, concerned about his health since a recent hospitalization, tries to keep him isolated from most inquiries about Entelev. His wife and children, however, seem to have taken a renewed interest in the product and imply that they may resume efforts to try to get it tested and approved.

192-1   (Re-typed copy)

cc: Chem. Dept. Files
    C.J.Lyons
    M.M.Baldwin
    G.A.Lutz
    PD Inf. Ctr.
    J.V.Sheridan
    R.S.Davidson
    Files

                                        January 7, 1963

Mr. W. A. Allen, Secretary
Else U. Pardee Foundation
923 West Park Drive
Midland, Michigan

Dear Mr. Allen:

     This is a follow up to our letter of March 26, 1962, and your
response of May 2, 1962, and concerns the hypothesis of Mr. Jim Sheridan.
At the time of our letter Jim had spent about six weeks with our staff.
Since our evaluation ultimately covered a ten-month period and was
recently completed, we are submitting this report designed to acquaint
you with the nature of our evaluation and to solicit your assistance in
carrying out our recommendations.

     In February 1962, it was our hope to complete our evaluation
in three months. Our first step was to set up a series of seminars as
well as meetings between Jim and each of about a dozen of our staff members - biochemists, biologists, physical chemists, cancer research people,
etc. The object of these meetings was to permit our staff members to
become completely conversant with Jims ideas. This approach ultimately
consumed five months and, frankly, was a failure. Our people seemed to
understand and receive favorably the broad concept, but the talks became
bogged down when detailed analysis of biochemical mechanisms was attempted.
We believe the failure to be caused by the fact that the hypothesis is
much too comprehensive for a specialist in a single discipline to follow
unless he can take considerable time to study the pertinent literature
of the several other disciplines involved.

     During the second five-month period we attempted to solve our
problems by providing a more concentrated effort by fewer people. Accordingly, two of our most competent biochemists spent the time necessary to
become completely familiar with the literature involved. Many lengthy
discussions were held during which all available data was interpreted
and discussed and during which possible routes of future experimentation
were explored.

     During this latter period we thought it wise to bring in outside
consultants and selected two men whom we believed to be uniquely qualified
to contribute to our study and discussions. Thus, you can see that we have
bent every effort to evaluate the hypothesis and to make an educated
judgement on its potential value for the future. *7/28/90*

Mr W.A.Allen   2   January 7, 1963

Our conclusions are:

1. The Sheridan hypothesis relating to the induction of tissue function,
   the influence of reversible chemical systems on tissue reversability,
   and the nature of a number of tissue abnormalities has a good proba-
   bility of being correct.

2. The hypothesis represents the best tool we know of for a breakthrough
   of major significance in our understanding of and control of cancer
   and perhaps a number of tissue abnormalities.

3. The hypothesis should lead us to a more complete understanding of many
   basic biological phenomenon - cell division, protein synthesis, tissue
   regeneration, wound healing, keloid scar formation, malignancy, and
   senescence.

4. The hypothesis, despite its comprehensive nature, is amenable to rather
   direct testing.

Our studies indicate that the future work should be divided into
several unit projects, each to be assigned to a team of qualified investiga
tors. Based on previous experience , we would expect each such unit to
cost §45,000 per year. Each unit would be completed in from two to three
years bringing the total cost of the projected program to about §300,000-
§500,000. It would be hoped to complete the entire program in three to
five years.

As you probably know, Battelle does not operate for profit and
therefor can carry only a small fraction of the financial burden for the
proposed work. We plan to solicit requests to government agencies and to
foundations like yours. In this connection we have already submitted one
such proposal to the Office of Naval Research.

It is our hope that you will support one of these unit projects
costing §45,000 per year. If, however, your commitments are such that you
cannot consider such a grant, we would appreciate your support of a portion
of one such unit. The funds will, of course, be accounted for, will be
administered by Battelle's administrative staff, and reports will be submitted periodically as the work proceeds.

We cordially invite you and your group to visit us here in
Columbus. If it will help you in any way, we will be pleased to send
several of our staff to Midland to discuss the proposed work with you.

We would like to comment on the real mystery behind the Sheridan
hypothesis. This is the disturbing question which occurs to everyone: "If
this is such a worthy idea, why has Jim failed to get all-out support durin
the many years he has been struggling with it?"

1/28/90

Mr. W. A. Allen   3   January 7, 1963

     The answer, of course, lies in the second question,"Why did it
take selected Battelle personnel ten months to reach the point of complete
comprehension of the hypothesis?". The hypothesis involves first an unorthodox approach to the study of tissue changes. We think it is unorthodox, but
believe it is sound. Secondly, interpretation of and implementation of the
hypothesis requires detailed and extensive background in an area in which
very few people have more than a general background. This area involves,
for example, the controlled shifting of the equilibrius position of a
reversable rate-limiting reaction as it occurs in cell division, not by the
usual mass action efforts, but by the chemical force resulting from the controlled shifting of the equilibrium position of a second reversible coupled
energy exchange reaction. It involves further a concept of how a specific
tissue function can be determined by the integrated rates of a number of
reversible chemical reactions.

     Cancer money has been spent in basic areas with the hope that
an accumulation of basic facts will someday suggest a reasonable unifying
theory. We have here not only a tool for basic research, but we have a
reasonable unifying theory. If we are to wait for the "simple" hypothesis
or a "chance" cure, we may wait forever. If the Sheridan hypothesis is
any criterion, and we believe it is, the hope for unifying theory will
not be "simple" and a chance cure is extremely remote.

     It is therefor easy to understand why foundations and experts
alike have been confused by and shunned support of this hypothesis. Under-
standably, they have not taken the time and effort to understand it or
evaluate it. Our decision then to take a leading role in a laboratory
implementation of the Sheridan hypothesis and to solicit the assistance
of others now stems from a deep conviction that this is not "just another"
proposal" but that this is an opportunity to provide a breakthrough in a
most perplexing disease.

                              Very truly yours

                              R. S. Davidson
                              Chief
                              Biosciences Research

I have read the above three (3)' pages and state that they are a faithful reproduction of a letter that I sent as Chief of Biosciences
Research at Battelle Columbus Laboratories.

     Date: _7/28/f0_____   _____

RSD/rdc

5
What Are Entelev and CanCell?

Jim Sheridan's The Technology of Entelev, IND-20258 and CanCell, an Identical Material, *Third Printing, November 1991. The new CanCell by Edward J. Sopcak.*

When Edward Sopcak took over the manufacturing and distribution of the material called Entelev from James Sheridan, he changed the name of the product he was producing to CanCell, but for a while the products remained identical. Then Sopcak began a gradual modification of the original formula and today's CanCell is quite different from the original Entelev. Sheridan, however, has made no changes in the original Entelev formula and he claims he has not manufactured it since stopping in 1983.

On June 15, 1992, Sopcak had printed a short note about an agreement to disassociate CanCell from Entelev reached by Sheridan's family and him on June 4, 1992. He now attaches this note to copies of *The Technology* whenever he gives it to anyone. See Document No. 8, page 90.

In order to fully explain his original hypothesis, Sheridan composed a detailed twenty-six-page accounting of his project in a booklet called *The Technology of Entelev, IND-20258 and CanCell, an Identical Material*, which he distributed free of charge to anyone who cared to read it. He encouraged people to copy and distribute it without charge in an effort to promote his ideas. It was composed when Entelev and CanCell were still identical materials. Pages 4, 8, and 20 were blank in the original document, so they appear as missing in many reproductions, but this is not an error of omission of any material. The blank pages usually are not reproduced. The entire document, minus the mentioned blank pages, is printed here as Document No. 9, page 91.

Sopcak believes this document graphically explains the way cells change when they become cancerous, and he makes it recommended reading for everyone who wants to understand how a normal cell changes to a cancer cell. Such patient education, providing detailed information describing how and why a disease causes illness, is practically unheard of in medical practice. Few drug companies bother to offer explanations to patients about how and why their products work. Physicians almost always give orders without explaining why. Both Sheridan and Sopcak respect the intelligence of patients and are eager to explain how and why they believe their products are successful.

When Sopcak began to modify the Entelev formula he was convinced that the success of the product was due to its energy that altered the vibrational frequencies of the cells, not just the chemistry of the compound. He believes that all allopathic medicines' effects are vibrational, not chemical as most pharmacists believe they are. As vibrational frequencies change, drugs become noneffective; physicians are unaware of or do not understand that hypothesis, although they are aware of drugs having a shelf life.

Every atom is really a galaxy of energy, and every compound is a combination of atoms, making a universe. Everything is energy, but that term will not satisfy biological scientists who demand exactness in an ever-changing energy situation that will never sustain exactness. Tradition-bound researchers simply cannot or will not understand this. They must be re-educated in the Electron Theory.

CanCell cures cancers by using a technology that exists but is not recognized or understood by very many scientists. When asked to explain how CanCell works, patients often reply that they don't care how it works; it just works and that is all they care about.

Several laboratories have tried to analyze CanCell but have been unable to do it and react by declaring it a fraud, just as they condemn anything they cannot understand. All of the chemicals in CanCell are on oxidation-reduction balance points and therefore the actual composition is variable according to atmospheric vibrations, which might be caused by temperature, light, location, etc. CanCell can't be analyzed because it keeps changing its energy. If scientists would take the time and effort to study and understand the Electron Theory and the relationship of energy and vibrational frequencies, as well as the killing and healing effects these have on cells, they would understand the cause of cancer and why CanCell cures it. The books listed in Chapter 1 make a good place to begin such an education.

The chemicals in CanCell have been chosen for their electrical properties. Their reaction with the body is electrical, not chemical. The material is nontoxic and it has no side effects. There have been over 30,000 animal tests done on Entelev and CanCell and it is estimated that between 10,000 and 12,000 people have taken it.

One of the most amazing parts of the CanCell story is that it is given free of charge to cancer patients. There is no charge for the material and there is no delivery charge, either. This is the only cancer treatment that has survived for over fifty years without some financial gain for someone. Nobody has made a profit from it. If this is not a valid, successful treatment, what has been the purpose for keeping it going? If Sheridan and Sopcak are quacks, what is their motive? It obviously has not been financial.

INFORMATION FOR THE FRIENDS AND USERS OF CANCELL AND/OR ENTELEV
AND FOR ALL THOSE WHO ARE INTERESTED IN THESE TECHNOLOGIES

On the fourth day of June, 1992, the Sheridan family, Mrs. Estelle, James E. Dennis and Margaret, but in the absence of James V. Sr., requested that my wife Gretchen and I meet with them, and we did.

The Sheridans requested that there be a separation of the Entelev technology. The viewpoint was expressed that this new improved CanCell was so different from the Entelev (1984 vintage) that James V. Sheridan Sr., with the concurrence of the Sheridan family, wished to have association with the new improved CanCell terminated.

It is felt that there is much merit in their viewpoint and therefore we agree with their request. The purpose of this release is to notify all who may be interested that the technology of CanCell has progressed to the point that it can no longer be explained using Jim Sheridan's "Technology of Entelev." However we believe that this paper should be studied. It is easily understood and will provide background for an understanding of the CanCell knowledge.

Edward J. Sopcak

June 15, 1992

The Technology of
ENTELEV, IND-20258
and
CANCELL,
an Identical Material

by
J. Sheridan

Third Printing, November 1991

Table of Contents

Abstract

CANCELL/ENTELEV are the products of an hypothesis. The *why* of its chemical make-up is answered by the hypothesis. The latter can be best explained by the use of a simplified cell model wherein there is set forth a definitive steady state for a hypothetical cell in

(a) its primitive state
(b) its differentiated state, and
(c) its malignant state.

1. In the model, the steady state of a normal cell (primitive form or differentiated form) comprises 12 energy units, $(ee-H^+)^{-1}$, per unit time flowing from a point of origin to a terminal acceptor.

2. In the case of the primitive form the 12 energy units all originate in glycolysis via the oxidation of glyceraldehyde phosphate.

   - The 12 $(ee-H^+)^{-1}$ are displaced from 12 glyceraldehyde phosphates by 12 phosphates $(P_i)^-$ which, in turn, are replaced by 12 $(OH)^-$ from 12 ADP; thus forming 12 ATP per unit time.

   - The 12 $(ee-H^+)^{-1}$ are picked up by NAD and then by pyruvate as the terminal acceptor.

   - This process requires the metabolism of 6 glucose molecules per unit time.

3. In the case of the differentiated cell the 12 $(ee-H^+)^{-1}$ have 6 different points of origin; that is, 2 $(ee-H^+)^{-1}$ from each point as follows:

pyruvate	$E_h = -0.60$ volt
ketoglutarate	$= -0.60$ volt
isocitrate	$= -0.30$ volt
glyceraldehyde	$= -0.28$ volt
malate	$= -0.17$ volt
succinate	$= -0.0$ volt
Average	$= -0.32$ volt

   - The 12 $(ee-H^+)^{-1}$ are picked up by respiratory enzymes and passed on stepwise to oxygen as the terminal acceptor.

   - This process requires 1 glucose molecule (glycolysis) and 6 HOH molecules (Krebs cycle) per unit time.

4. In the case of the cancer cell the steady state of $(ee-H^+)^{-1}$ flow to terminal acceptors is the sum of the primitive form and the differentiated form. Thus, in unit time, we have the following:

   A. 7 glucose molecules metabolizing with 12 $(ee-H^+)^{-1}$ going to pyruvate as the terminal acceptor and 6 $(ee-H^+)^{-1}$ going to oxygen as the terminal acceptor.

   B. 6 HOH molecules entering the Krebs cycle with 6 $(ee-H^+)^{-1}$ going to oxygen as the terminal acceptor.

5. In the differentiated cell a normal chemical work demand on the ATP inventory leads to a manageable decease in ATP and a manageable increase in P_i and ADP. The increase in ADP effects an increased rate of flow of $(ee-H^+)^{-1}$.

6. The increase in rate of flow of $(ee-H^+)^{-1}$ causes a decrease in the AV. between cyt.b and cyt.c. The AV.between cyt.b and cyt.c. will be referred to as the "cyt.b. valve".

   • At the same time the increase in P_i and ADP causes an increase in the rate of $(ee-H^+)^{-1}$ production in glycolysis; that is, in the rate of replacement of $(ee-H^+)^{-1}$ by P_i from glyceraldehyde phosphate. The resulting increased rate of flow of the latter $(ee-H^+)^{-1}$ to NAD will result in a relatively larger reduction of NAD (a lowering of the redox potential of the NAD-NADH system). The up-and-down movement of the NAD-NADH redox potential will be referred to as the "glycolysis valve".

7. If the work demand on ATP in the differentiated cell is large enough to be unmanageable and chronic, the following occurs:

   A. The rate of $(ee-H^+)^{-1}$ flow through the cyt.b.-cyt.c. crossover point increases to a point where the AV. between cyt.b. and cyt.c. becomes too small (less than about 0.18 volt) to supply the energy (about 8.3 Kcal.) necessary for ATP formation. As a result, this crossover point becomes uncoupled from phosphorylation. For this reason the cyt.b. valve is said to be "closed" to phosphorylation. In this manner the production of 12 ATP molecules per unit time is being lost and the concentrations of P_i and ADP increases accordingly. This is one of the 2 initial steps of carcinogenesis.

   B. As a result of the increased availability of P_i and ADP there is an increase in the rate of production of $(ee-H^+)^{-1}$ in glycolysis and the rate of flow of $(ee-H^+)^{-1}$ from glyceraldehyde phosphate to NAD becomes rapid enough to reduce the redox potential of the NAD-NADH system to a point below the redox potential of the pyruvate-lactate system. This results in an increased rate of flow of $(ee-H^+)^{-1}$ to pyruvate and the glycolysis valve is said to be "open" to pyruvate as a terminal acceptor. This is also one of the 2 initial steps of carcinogenesis.

   C. If the cyt.b. valve is closed and the glycolysis valve is open, the process starts to move toward a point of irreversibility.

   D. The point of irreversibility is reached when 7 molecules of glucose are being metabolized per unit time (the steady state of a cancer cell having been reached).

8. The suggested treatment for cancer is to change the steady state of cancer to the steady state of the primitive cell. The suggested method involves:

A. Blocking the energy unit from flowing through the cytochrome system. By way of example, the reduced form of catechol blocks between cyt.b. and cyt.c.

B. Shunting the blocked energy units directly to a terminal acceptor. Preferred sites for picking up the energy units are:

   1. At or just above $+0.29$ volt the $\acute{E}_o$ of cyt.a, to intercept units which have escaped the catechol block and are entering the highest crossover point for ATP formation.

   2. At about $E_h = -0.17$ to -0.21 volt, the redox level of the cancer cell.

   3. Immediately above 0.0 volt, the $\acute{E}_o$ of succinate oxidation, the highest voltage of entrance of $(ee\text{-}H^+)^{-1}$ into the respiration system.

   4. Just above -0.28 volt; that is, about -0.25 to -0.28 volt; to intercept the 8 $(ee\text{-}H^+)^{-1}$ entering the respiratory system at or below that point.

   5. At $E_h = -0.32$ volt, the half wave potential of the NAD $\rightleftharpoons$ NADH system.

   6. At, or near, $E_h = -0.6$ volt - the most reduced O-R level of the Krebs cycle.

Background

Warburg, during his extensive studies on respiratory activity in the cancer cell, paid considerable attention to the relatively high rate of glycolysis of cancer tissue. As a result of this he suggested that carcinogenesis resulted from a chronic lack of energy in the normal cell.

Initially Warburg thought that the "lack of energy" was a result of "damage" to the respiratory system with a resulting lowering in the quantity of ATP being produced. The "low production" idea didn't prove out. Warburg, however, still sensing a problem with ATP, suggested that the ATP produced in fermentation (glycolysis) might be different from the ATP in normal respiration—perhaps different in that it was made in a different geographical zone in the cell.

Warburg also concluded:

1. Cancer cells have "high fermentation values—very close to those of wildly proliferating Torula yeasts".

2. That we will understand the origin of "cancer" when we know how this high fermentation rate originates".

3. That, in cancer cells, respiration has been "damaged" and this, in some manner, is related to the origin of the high fermentation rate (high glycolytic rate).

4. That the "damage" to respiration may be caused by the "breaking of the coupling between respiration and the formation of ATP".

5. That the action of the carcinogenic "agent" must be chronic and the "damage" must be irreversible.

I agree with these numbered conclusions and, if they are true, we are left with the questions:

1. What is the nature of the alleged "damage"?

2. How does the "damage" initiate an increase in "fermentation"?

3. Why is the "damage" irreversible?

4. How is the shift from a Pasteur effect to a Crabtree effect accounted for?

5. How is the high glycolytic rate of some normal tissues accounted for?

Such a quick acceptance of the essential correctness of Warburg's perception of carcinogenesis immediately raises a question.

Query: If Warburg was essentially correct in his perception of carcinogenesis, why—35 years later—has science failed to build on that perception to the point of a generally acceptable hypothesis explaining carcinogenesis?

Answer: The problem does not lie in what Warburg, and seemingly everyone else, has been discussing, but, rather in an item that is not being discussed.

Otto Warburg—On the Origin of Cancer Cells
Science Vol. 123 No. 3191 2-24-56)

The Problem

When Warburg and the others discussed "energy" they became mired down in discussions about ATP to the almost complete exclusion of other energy units and, particularly, to the exclusion of the equilibria between these units.

The reason for such exclusion appears to be that no one has yet suggested a "generic" energy unit which can be used to define the steady state of (for example) a primitive tissue, a differentiated tissue, and a malignant tissue—and how a tissue might move from one such steady state to another to:

    (a) cause a cancer, or

    (b) to cure a cancer.

The hypothesis to be discussed herein defines such an energy unit, defines the steady state referred to, and defines a possible pathway from one such steady state to another.

Query: Taking into account the energy unit, $(ee\text{-}H^+)^{-1}$; was Warburg correct in suspecting that there is a difference between (a) ATP made in glycolysis and (b) ATP made in respiration?

Answer: Yes, Warburg was correct. There are at least 2 very significant differences.:

    1.(a) In glycolysis the reaction that produces $(ee\text{-}H^+)^{-1}$ *also* produces ATP.

       (b) However, in respiration ATP is made at the expense of $(ee\text{-}H^+)^{-1}$ energy.

    2.(a) The system making glycolytic ATP in response to a work demand—by producing $(ee\text{-}H^+)^{-1}$ at a low redox potential —delivers $(ee\text{-}H^+)^{-1}$ to NAD and thus tends to reduce the NAD-NADH system.

       (b) However, the system making respiratory ATP in response to a work demand—increases the rate of flow of $(ee\text{-}H^+)^{-1}$ and hence tends to *oxidize* the NAD-NADH system.

The importance of these differences will be discussed.

Chance and Williams reported an analog computer representation of a five-membered oxidative phosphorylation chain acting according to the law of mass action. The changes in the steady-state oxidation-reduction levels were measured following an addition of ADP.

    Note: The addition of ADP is considered here as simulating a chemical work demand on ATP which would also result in an increase in ADP.

The results show an oxidation of NADH and cyt.b and a reduction of cyt.c, cyt.a, and cyt.a$_3$. The oxidation of cyt.b together with the reduction of cyt.c effects a reduction in the ΔV. between the 2 enzymes.

This subject matter was also reviewed quite extensively by Klingenberg. In his Figure 15, for example, he shows the effect of adding ATP to the active state of mitochondria. the effect being the opposite of adding ADP relative to the response of cyt.b and cyt.c.

Chance and Williams: Advances in Enzymology 17 p. 56 (1956)

M. Klingenberg: Biological Oxidations, Interscience Publishers
      Edited by T.C. Singer (1968)

Figure 15 of Klingenberg shows the degree of reduction of cyt.b changing from about 14% to about 56% (Δ 42%) while cyt.c went from about 26% to about 40% (Δ 14%). Thus, the addition of ATP (satisfying a work demand) increases the ΔV. of the cyt.b-cyt.c crossover point while the addition of ADP (simulating an increased work demand) *decreases* the ΔV.

Query: Why is it important to note this particular deviation of cyt.b from the response of the other cytochromes?

Answer: Because a normal cell under an unusually large work demand could:

(a) respond with a sufficient lowering of the ΔV. at the cyt.b-cyt.c crossover point to uncouple the point from phosphorylation, and

(b) consequently, put an abnormal work demand on the glycolytic system, and

(c) consequently, shift the steady state of the system from normal to cancer.

The Energy Unit

The energy unit of the cell model can be symbolized as:

$$(ee\text{-}X^+)^{-1}$$

It exists as a univalent negative grouping or as a univalent negative radical. It comprises:

A. 2 covalent electrons (ee) which carry the energy.

B. a positive charge (X^+) which can be:

    1. A proton. For example, in the hydride ion:

    $H^{-1} = (ee\text{-}H^+)^{-1}$

    or in the hydroxyl ion:

    $(OH)^- = (O^o\text{-}ee\text{-}H^+)^{-1}$

    2. The positive grouping from a phosphate ion:

    $(O^o\text{-}PO_3H_2{}^+)^{-1} = (O^o\text{-}ee\text{-}PO_3H_2{}^+)^{-1}$

    3. The positive grouping from ADP:

$$\begin{array}{cc} O & O \\ \| & \| \\ HO\text{-}P\text{-}O\text{-}P\text{-}OR \\ | & | \\ OH & OH \end{array} = (H^+\text{-}ee\text{-}O^o)^{-1}\text{-}P_2O_6H_2R^+$$

    or as it appears in ATP:

$$(RH_2O_6P_2{}^+\text{-}ee\text{-}O^o)^{-1}\text{-}PO_3H_2{}^+$$

Discussion of The Energy Unit

The structure of HOH, a polar molecule, is usually shown as follows:

$$\begin{array}{ccc} H & & H \\ \diagdown & & \diagup \\ & O & \end{array}$$

or, to emphasize the polarity and the importance of the 2 electrons derived from the hydrogen atoms:

The nature of the bond between one of the protons and the electron pair (ee) can be altered by:

1. Removing the other proton as in ionization (see Figure 1).

2. Putting energy into the molecule as in electrolysis and photosynthesis (see Figure 1).

It is important to note that in ionization and in photosynthesis the right sides (as shown) of the structures have been reduced; that is, gained in energy by the movement of the electrons relative to the remaining H^+.

This same phenomenon occurs in the formulation of ATP and in the utilization of ATP in the doing of chemical work.

FIGURE 1

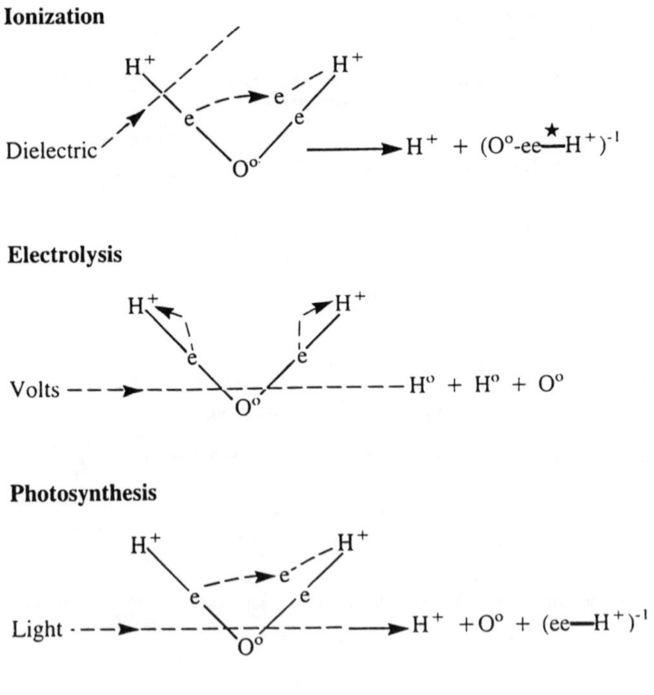

Ionization

Electrolysis

Photosynthesis

★ The — is a relatively strong bond.

This is shown in Figure 2—the Formation of ATP in Glycolysis. The figure shows the oxidation of glyceraldehyde phosphate to phosphoglyceric acid in the following steps:

1. Phosphate (P_i) oxidizes the aldehyde by replacing the hydrogen atom. The latter is in the form of the energy unit, $(ee\text{-}H^+)^{-1}$ and enters the respiratory system by transfer to NAD.

2. The $(OH)^{-1}$ of ADP replaces the P_i to form the acid. Simultaneously, the bond between the P and the OH of ADP is broken which permits the P_i to replace the OH from ADP.

It is submitted that the most significant step here is the breaking of the ADP to $(OH)^-$ bond. This step makes possible the replacement by P_i and the shift of (ee) from P_i to ADP. It will be seen that a similar event occurs in respiration except that there is a $(ee\text{-}H^+)^{-1}$ which breaks the bond.

Figure 3—Formation of ATP—Respiration shows the transfer of energy from a $(ee\text{-}H^+)^{-1}$ moving through a voltage gradient in the following steps:

1. The $(ee\text{-}H^+)^{-1}$ leaves the enzyme at the bottom of the drawing and moves toward the enzyme near the top of the drawing. It contacts ADP and breaks the ADP-OH bond. Since the ADP picks up the energy it is acting as an oxidizing agent.

2. The $(ee\text{-}H^+)^{-1}$ is replaced by P_i (again, as in glycolysis, acting as an oxidizing agent) to form ATP.

FIGURE 2

Formation of ATP in Glycolysis

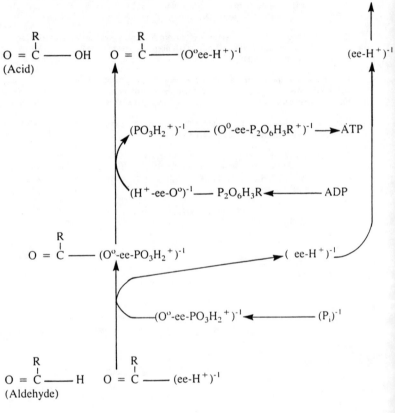

FIGURE 3

Formation of ATP—Respiration

$(ee-H^+)^{-1}$ moving through a voltage gradient

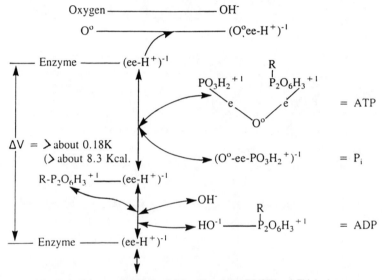

Again, it is submitted the most significant step is breaking of the ADP-OH bond. This leads to the combination of ADP and $(ee-H^+)^{-1}$, then the combination of ADP and P_i. Again a shift of (ee) from P_i to ADP occurs.

Figure 4—Chemical Work by ATP—illustrates the transfer of energy by using, for example, the formation of a peptide bond in the following steps:

1. The $PO_3H_2^+$ grouping of the ATP breaks the bond between the OH and carbon of an amino acid and combines with OH to reform P_i.

2. The $(P_2O_6H_2R^+-ee-O^o)^{-1}$ grouping of ATP breaks the bond between the nitrogen and hydrogen of a second amino acid and combines with the H^+ to reform ADP.

FIGURE 4

**Chemical Work By ATP—
Formation of a Peptide Bond**

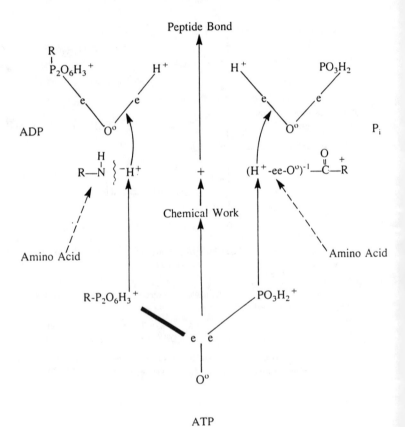

The Steady State

In the cell model (whether primitive, differentiated or cancer) the steady state is defined as:

The movement of 12 (ee-H$^+$)$^{-1}$ per unit time through a voltage gradient to a terminal acceptor. Only the terminal acceptor(s) changes.

Primitive is 12 (ee-H$^+$)$^{-1}$ per unit time moving from NADH to pyruvate.

Differentiated is 12 (ee-H$^+$)$^{-1}$ per unit time moving from cyt.b to oxygen via the cytochrome system.

Cancer is 12 (ee-H$^+$)$^{-1}$ per unit time moving from NADH to pyruvate *and* 12 (ee-H$^+$)$^{-1}$ per unit time moving from cyt.b to oxygen.

The difference between the primitive and differentiated states is established by the position of glycolysis valve—*open* in a primitive cell and *closed* in a differentiated cell.

The difference between the differentiated and cancer steady states is established by the positions of 2 valves—a glycolysis valve and a cyt.b valve.

	glycolysis valve	cyt.b valve
differentiated cell	closed	open
cancer cell	open	closed

The Glycolysis Valve

In the cell model the critical parameter which separates the primitive steady state from the differentiated steady state is the redox level of the NAD-NADH system relative to the redox level of the pyruvate-lactate system (see Figure 5).

In the primitive cell the NAD-NADH level is lower than the pyruvate-lactate level and the flow of (ee-H$^+$)$^{-1}$ is from the former to the latter. The valve is *open*.

In the differentiated cell the NAD-NADH level is higher than the pyruvate-lactate level, the valve is *closed*, and there is no flow of (ee-H$^+$)$^{-1}$ to pyruvate.

Cyt.b Valve

The cyt.b valve operates in response to the voltage difference (ΔV.) between cyt.b and cyt.c.

The equilibrium redox levels of cyt.b and cyt.c are about +0.08 volt and +0.26 volt, respectively—a ΔV. of 0.18 volt. An energy unit moving through 0.18 volt can transfer about 8.3 Kcal. per mol. The latter figure is used in the cell model.

In other words, if the ΔV. in the cyt.b-cyt.c crossover point drops below about 0.18 volt, and ATP molecule cannot form (see Figure 6).

Page 15

Chance and Williams, as pointed out above, have shown that adding ADP (a) increases the rate of flow of energy units; (b) increases the relative rate of oxidation of NADH, flavins, and cyt.b; and increases the relative rate of reduction of cyt.c and cyt.a. The oxidation of cyt.b and the reduction of cyt.c decreases the ΔV. of the crossover point between them.

Therefore, if the ΔV. of the cyt.b valve is less than 0.18 volt in the cell model, the crossover point is *closed* to phosphorylation (i.e. uncoupled). Such a closing, at a steady state, means the loss of 12 ATP per unit time at the cyt.b-cyt.c crossover.

Figure 5

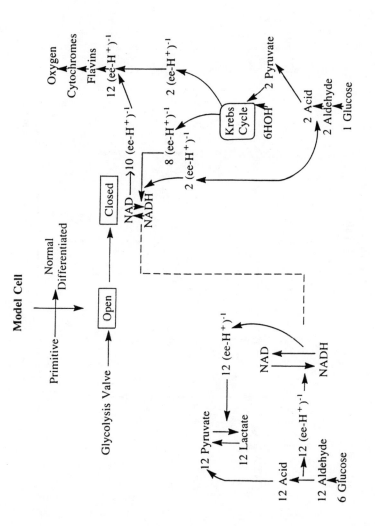

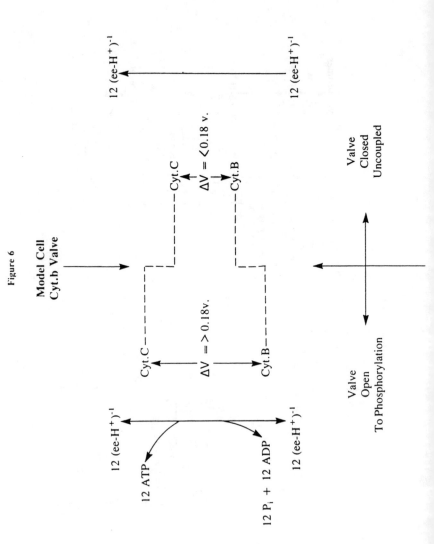

Figure 6

Work Demand—An Example

Using the formation of peptides or protein (P) from amino acids (A) we have:

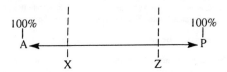

Where X is the true equilibrium position of the system and Z is a desired steady state position necessary for P to perform some necessary function.

To get from X to Z, and maintain it at Z, requires chemical work (ΔF). ATP can do such work by a transfer of energy (-ΔF).

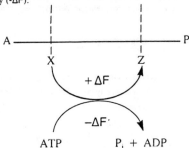

Thus, the system A——▶P is making a *work demand* on the ATP system.

Carcinogenesis

It is a common conception that "cancer is 100 diseases with 100 causes". The hypothesis proposed here is a complete departure from this idea. A second common conception is that cancer results from some untoward change in the genes. I would restate this as "There is an untoward change in the genes which results from the *single* cause of the disease".

1. Cancer is one disease with one cause.

2. The cause is a chronic, abnormal, chemical work demand which affects the steady state of a differentiated cell by a definable shift in energy supply—

    (a) from a crossover point (cyt.b-cyt.c) where ATP energy is being *increased* at the expense of a *decreasing* energy in $(ee\text{-}H^+)^{-1}$ units moving through the respiratory voltage gradient—

    (b) to a point where ATP is being produced jointly with $(ee\text{-}H^+)^{-1}$; that is, ATP energy and $(ee\text{-}H^+)^{-1}$ energy are *both being increased* —the cost being an increased glucose metabolism (glycolysis).

A pertinent question at this point is:

Query: If—

    (a) the cell is under an increasing work demand, and

    (b) consequently the rate of usage of ATP is increasing, and

    (c) consequently, the rate of production of P_i and ADP is increasing, and

    (d) consequently, the rate of production of $(ee\text{-}H^+)^{-1}$ in glycolysis is increasing, and

    (e) consequently, the rate of movement of $(ee\text{-}H^+)^{-1}$ through the cytochrome system is increasing

    —is there a limit to this escalation?

Answer: Yes.

As indicated above (and as suspected by Warburg), the cell has a reserve scheme whereby it can effect a large increase in available free energy by moving toward a new steady state. Unfortunately (and as suspected by Warburg), the new steady state is cancer.

The steps of the shift are as follows (see Figure 8):

Step 1

Starting in the model with a differentiated cell in the controlled state,

    (a) there are 12 $(ee\text{-}H^+)^{-1}$ units per unit time moving through the cytochrome system to oxygen.

Page 21

(b) the ΔV. of the cyt.b-cyt.c valve is at least 0.18 volt—the valve is *open* to phosphorylation.

(c) 1 molecule of glucose per unit time is metabolizing.

(d) the flow of $(ee-H^+)^{-1}$ from glyceraldehyde phosphate to NAD-NADH is acting to *reduce* the latter and the flow from NAD-NADH to oxygen is acting to *oxidize* the latter at a steady state rate which poises the redox potential of NAD-NADH above that of pyruvate-lactate—the glycolysis valve is *closed*.

Figure 7

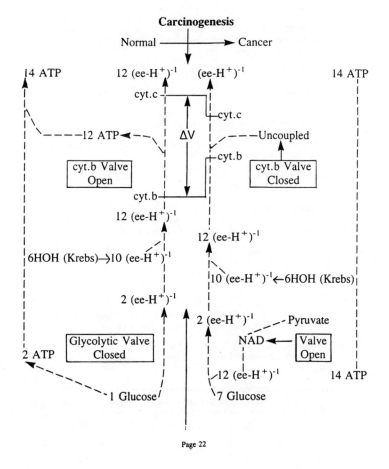

Page 22

Step 2

The cell of the model is subjected to a normal, relatively small work demand.

    (a) The rate of usage of ATP increases and, consequently, the concentrations of P_i and ADP increase.

    (b) Consequently, in glycolysis, the rate of reaction of glyceraldehyde phosphate to phosphoglyceric acid increases and the rate of metabolism of glucose increases.

    (c) Consequently, the rate of production of $(ee\text{-}H^+)^{-1}$ increases but not enough to lower the NAD-NADH sufficiently to close the glycolysis valve.

    (d) Consequently, the rate of movement of $(ee\text{-}H^+)^{-1}$ through the cytochrome system increases but not enough to lower the AV. of the cyt.-b-cyt.c crossover point sufficiently to open the cyt.b valve.

Step 3

The work demand on the cell of the model becomes larger and chronic.

    (a) The rate of usage of ATP increases even more, and consequently, the concentrations of P_i and ADP increase even more.

    (b) Consequently, in glycolysis, the rate of reaction of aldehyde to acid increases and the rate of metabolism of glucose increases.

    (c) Consequently, the rate of production of $(ee\text{-}H^+)^{-1}$ increases but still *not enough to open* the glycolysis valve.

    (d) The rate of movement of $(ee\text{-}H^+)^{-1}$ through the cyt.b-cyt.c crossover point now reaches a level where the AV. is reduced to less than 0.18 volt. The cyt.b valve *closes* and the crossover point is uncoupled from phosphorylation.

    (e) The Pasteur effect has been lifted.

Step 4

As a consequence of Step 3:

    (a) The step of uncoupling from phosphorylation releases a "flood" 'of P_i and ADP which was being used in the cyt.b-cyt.c crossover point.

    (b) Consequently, the flood of P_i and ADP has a comparatively great effect on the rate of the aldehyde-acid reaction and there is a large increase in $(ee\text{-}H^+)^{-1}$ production.

    (c) Consequently, the increase in $(ee\text{-}H^+)^{-1}$ is large enough to reduce the NAD-NADH redox level to that of the pyruvate-lactate; thus *closing* the glycolysis valve. With this valve closed the Crabtree effect is in operation.

Page 23

(d) Consequently, the rate of glucose metabolism increases until 6 additional molecules per unit time are being metabolized—which means 12 $(ee-H^+)^{-1}$ per unit time are moving to pyruvate.

(e) Consequently, the cell has moved to the new steady state—cancer.

(f) Consequently, 12 additional ATP molecules per unit time are being produced in glycolysis, which equals the 12 lost in respiration.

The Selected Chemicals

The *system* of chemicals selected must mimic the oxidation-reduction character of the natural system. However, it must shift the steady state characteristic of a cancer cell to a steady state characteristic of a primitive cell.

Thus, if a perfect result were achieved in the cell model the result would be:

1. The 12 $(ee\text{-}H^+)^{-1}$ moving from cyt.b to oxygen would be reduced to zero. This would require:

   A. The flow of $(ee\text{-}H^+)^{-1}$ through the cytochrome system must be blocked, or

   B. the flow must be *shunted* to a terminal acceptor other than oxygen, or

   C. A combination of *both* of the above. The combination is expected to be more effective because the shunting of a substantial proportion of $(ee\text{-}H^+)^{-1}$ takes the "pressure" off the blocker so that it is relatively more effective.

2. Some of the $(ee\text{-}H^+)^{-1}$ in the primitive system will be shunted to a terminal acceptor—the degree of this shunting to be determined by empirical methods. This for the reason that the uncoupling of the entire cytochrome system might cause too great a response from the primitive system.

The Selection

Catechol is a known blocker—blocking between cyt.b and cyt.c

The ortho-quinone form is a known shunter—shunting electrons directly to oxygen.

Caution: The para-quinones are also good shunters except they deliver electrons back into the cytochrome system. For example: α-tocopheral oxide (from vitamin E) and coenzyme Q.

Ascorbic acid, although not a quinone, also shunts electrons into the cytochrome system. This property is involved in the oxidation of proline to hydroxy proline—which leads to the *formulation of excessive collage* and may be presumed to be involved in *protein formation in the Aids virus.*

A second characteristic of a selected chemical (in addition to being a catechol) is that it has a redox potential at a selected level. Particularly important levels are:

1. Immediately above cyt.a to pick up $(ee\text{-}H^+)^{-1}$ entering the crossover point above cyt.a. Catechols with half-wave potentials about cyt.a will be substantially reduced at tissue potential level and can function as blockers.

2. The redox level of the cancer cell.

A third important characteristic is the compound's pK levels.

Protocol For CanCell

*Sopcak prescribes a holistic approach. Life style
and diet changes. How to order CanCell.*

Edward Sopcak claims that about 80 percent of all cancer patients who use CanCell become clinically free of the disease. Those who do not, he speculates, fail because they do not follow the prescribed holistic protocol, along with using the material as directed; or the vibrational frequency may have been altered by improper storage, such as placing it near an electrical outlet, rendering it useless. He has developed what he calls a new improved formula, which he describes in a pamphlet that he sends along with instructions in every supply he gives, free of charge, to patients. The new CanCell is delivered in two bottles, labeled C and G, along with individual calibrated plastic droppers to measure dosages. The following is a re-typed copy of the latest insert, printed here as Document No. 10.:

<u>IMPORTANT INFORMATION ABOUT CANCELL</u>
May 19, 1992

WHAT IS CANCELL?
CanCell is an assembly of synthetic chemicals. There is nothing natural in the product. These chemicals are created for their electrical properties. CanCell reacts with the body electrically, therefore it is nontoxic and it has no side effects.

CanCell lowers the voltage of the cell structure of the body by about 20%. That is significant for the following reason: all cancer is a mutation of anaerobic cells, or cells which do not use oxygen to create energy.

Because these anaerobic cells are weak cells, they lyse or convert directly to waste material when voltage is lowered. This is also true of the protein coating on the HIV and other viruses.

The cancer cells are not killed and they do not die. They simply digest. The waste material from this digestion has the appearance of raw egg whites. The body eliminates this waste material any way it can. It can appear in the urine, the stool, or as vaginal discharge. It may be thrown up or coughed up and it may be eliminated in perspiration. Any, all, or none of these may happen. The cancer cells are replaced with normal oxygen-using cells and the cancer cells no longer exist.

PLEASE READ THESE
DIRECTIONS IMMEDIATELY!

STORAGE OF CANCELL

• Keep in drawer or closet.
• Do not allow the bottles to touch each other. If you must transport them out of the house, place each bottle in a separate sock.
• Do not place these bottles near any electrical appliance, outlet, microwave, television, radio, refrigerator, electric blanket, or digital clock.
• Do not expose to x-rays in an airport.

USE OF CANCELL C AND G

USE FORMULAS C AND G INTERNALLY

Take every 12 hours as follows: wait at least 20 minutes after eating or drinking before you take these formulas. Shake each bottle before using. In any order, put ½ (0.5) cc under your tongue and wait five minutes before you swallow. Then do the same with the other formula. Wait at least 20 minutes before eating or drinking again. Never take these formulas rectally.

ALSO USE FORMULA C EXTERNALLY

Use every 12 hours as follows: shake Formula C and use for patches. Every 12 hours apply ½ (0.5) cc to a small, flat cotton cosmetic pad. Tape pad below the crease on the inside of the elbow with waterproof tape. Cover it completely so that it will not dry out. You <u>do not</u> need to use DMSO.

WARNINGS

• If you are on diabetes medication you must monitor your blood sugar carefully. Late-onset diabetes leaves the body at the same time that cancer does.

WHAT YOU CAN EXPECT
WHILE TAKING CANCELL

There are no side effects to taking CanCell; however, your body will be eliminating toxic waste material from the cancer and other waste breakdown products. This discharge can cause flu-like symptoms, loss of energy, and weakness. These symptoms are part of the healing process and are temporary. The elimination of this waste material is a very important part of the CanCell program.

TO IMPROVE ELIMINATION

• VEGETARIAN DIET. Eat raw fruits and vegetables, preferably organic. Juicing is recommended, especially when the cancer involves any of the digestive organs. Do not eat meat, sugar, dairy products, alcohol, and caffeine. Sugar can stop the effects of CanCell. Note: If you are using CanCell for MS, request additional dietary suggestions.

• DISTILLED WATER. Drink 64-128 ounces (8 16-ounce glasses) each day. Distilled water (not reverse-osmosis water) is the only water that is negatively charged. This negative charge will attract waste material and help carry it out of the body.

• BROMELAIN (an enzyme from pineapple). This should be used by everyone who uses CanCell. Take at least 1,000 mg. before or with each meal. Use a total of at least 3,000 mg per day.

• GLUTATHIONE (an amino acid to support cleansing of the liver). Only to be used by those who have liver cancer, AIDS, or herpes viruses. Take at least 1,000 mg. of glutathione before or with each meal.

• BHT (Butalated Hydroxy Toluline). Only to be used if you have AIDS or herpes. Take 2,000 mg. of BHT on an empty stomach before retiring each night.

• WILLARD'S WATER (a lignite-activated water which assists in the assimilation of nutrients and in the discharge of waste material from the lymphatic system). Add 2 ounces to each gallon of distilled water.

• BOWEL MOVEMENT. It is extremely important to keep your bowels moving. To keep toxic waste from building up in your system, do any or all of these: 1. Use plenty of raw fruit and raw fruit juices (they stimulate the bowels); 2. Use a good herbal laxative, if necessary; 3. Enemas and/or colonic baths are recommended, if needed.

• THE ABOVE ITEMS can be found at your local health food store. For your convenience, bromelain, glutathione, BHT and Willard's Water are also available from Nutrition Hotline. However, CanCell is to be used immediately. Do not wait until you get bromelain, glutathion or BHT.

CANCELL CANNOT BE USED WITH. . .

• Mint. This includes toothpaste, tea, mouthwash. (You can use baking soda and salt for toothpaste or Tom's Fennel Toothpaste from the health food store.)

• Any other cancer or AIDS therapy. This includes chemotherapy, radiation, hormone therapy, AZT, DDI, acupuncture, Rife, or other vibrational therapies, radionics ozone or other oxygen therapies, etc.

• Nicotine in the blood from any source.

• Any vitamin, mineral or herbal supplement. CanCell lowers voltage of the cells while vitamins, herbs, minerals,and homeopathic remedies raise the energy of the cells. They will conflict.

- Electric blankets. Do not sleep under an electric blanket.

IT IS UNDERSTOOD

- CanCell is not approved by the FDA or AMA.
- It is provided under common law principle. The use or acceptance of CanCell is evidence of your acceptance of the common law and/or the U.S. Constitutional law.
- CanCell was requested by you, and no claims are made for CanCell.
- The decision to take CanCell is solely yours.

PLEASE NOTE

- The request for CanCell must be made verbally by the person who intends to use it.
- Our ability to provide CanCell is limited; therefore, do not request CanCell unless you intend to use it. There are many others to whom it may be a matter of life or death.
- CanCell is a rare material and should never be misused or wasted. By requesting it, it is assumed that you agree to follow the program as directed.

WHEN TO REORDER

These formulas last approximately 52 days if taken as directed. Send in your reorder form no earlier than 30 days and no later than 40 days from the day you begin. Only reorder if the symptoms are still present, except with the AIDS virus. Research indicates that the AIDS virus is eliminated in 28 days.

FOR MORE INFORMATION

- AUDIO TAPES are available from Nutrition Hotline, P.O. Box 840, Milford, MI 48381-0840. $10,00 each.
    CanCell: What it is, What it does
    CanCell: Dietary Recommendations
    CanCell Update. 1992 Global Science Congress

- VIDEO TAPES are also available from Nutrition Hotline, P.O. Box 840, Milford, MI 48381-0840. $25.00 each.

CanCell Update, 1992 Global Science Congress
Testimonial, At Whose Expense

• DOCTOR'S INFORMATION can be requested on the physician's letterhead. This is a package containing more technical information about CanCell.

• QUESTIONS AND CORRESPONDENCE should be directed to Vibrational Research Foundation, P.O. Box 265, Milford, MI 48381-0265.

• REQUESTS FOR CanCell should be directed to The Volunteer Request Line, 11:00 A.M. to 3:00 P.M. (Eastern Time), Monday through Friday at (313) 684-5529. No calls are accepted Saturday, Sunday or holidays. The phone line is very busy; you must be persistent and use your redial.

• TERMINAL PATIENTS only may request CanCell in writing but the following requirements must be met.
    1. The terminal patient must have read the information on the use of CanCell and must state in their letter that they are informed and wish to use CanCell. They must also include their name, address, phone number, age, date of original diagnosis, treatments used, and current medications in use.
    2. The above letter must be accompanied by a letter of prognosis from the doctor. A prognosis states the condition of the patient and his/her life expectancy. This letter must be on the doctor's letterhead and signed by the doctor. We cannot accept a diagnosis or medical records. Send these mail requests to P.O. Box 265, Milford, MI 48381.

• CANCELL IS IN EXTREMELY LIMITED SUPPLY but MAY be available for the following conditions by special request: ALS (Lou Gehrig's disease), Multiple Sclerosis, Muscular Dystrophy, Parkinson's, Alzheimer's, Scleroderma, EXTREME cases of emphysema and diabetes, and certain VERY RARE maladies. These requests must be made by phone.

* * * *

Sopcak makes dietary recommendations that he sends along with each supply of CanCell. A re-typed copy is printed here as Document No. 11:

DIETARY RECOMMENDATIONS

Ideal Diet

Note: There is no limit on quantities of these foods. It is best to eat them all day long.
- **Organic Raw Fruits & Juices**
- **Organic Raw Vegetables & Juices**
- **Sprouts** of any kind—Alfalfa, Mung bean, Radish Seed, Lentils, Peas, Garbanzo beans, Sunflower Seeds, Buckwheat, etc.
- **Distilled Water**

Foods acceptable in Limited Quantity

These are listed in descending order, starting with the most acceptable.
- **Raw Seeds and Nuts**
- **Dried Fruit**—sundried only, no sulfurdioxide
- **Steamed Organic Vegetables**
- **Tempeh and Organic Tofu**
- **Cold Pressed Oils**—imported olive oils or any Spectrum Natural brand oil, Flora brand, or Arrowhead Mills brand. Refrigerate after opening. No supermarket oils.
- **Shellfish**—Shrimp, Crab, Lobster, Oysters, Clams, etc.
- **Ocean Fish**—Prepared any way except fried.
- **Grains**—Brown Rice, Wheat, Rye, Oats, Buckwheat, Barley, Millet, Amaranth, Quinoa, Corn, Teff, etc.
- **Foods made from grains**: Pastas and Breads—whole grain varieties only. No refined white flour.
- **Beans, Peas and Legumes**—Pinto, Navy, White, Black, Kidney, Garbanzo, Azuki, Soy, Lima, Lentil, Peanuts, etc.
- **Herbs and Spices**—Herb teas: Only Peppermint, Spearmint and Chamomile; Other herbs may interfere.
- **Natural Sweeteners**—Honey, Barley Malt, Rice Syrup, Maple Syrup, Concentrated Fruit Juices, etc.

Foods Extremely Limited
• **Chicken, Turkey, Duck, or other Game, and Eggs:** These can only be consumed if you are sure that they have been grown without growth hormones, antibiotics, steroids, arsenic, etc.
• **Caffeine**
• **Alcohol**

Foods Never to Eat
• **Red Meat**—Beef, Pork, Lamb, Sausage, Hotdogs, Ham, Bacon Lunchmeats, etc.
• **Dairy Products**—Milk, Ice Cream, Sour Cream, Cheese, Butter, Cottage Cheese, Yogurt, Non-Fat Dried Milk, etc. Watch Labels. Also watch Gravies, Salad Dressings and Creamed Soups.
• **Hydrogenated Oils**—Margarine and oils used in most boxed foods. Read Labels.
• ****White Sugar****—Sucrose, Dextrose, Maltose, Corn Syrup, Fructose, etc. Watch pop, candy, cookies, pies, cakes, etc.
• **Artificial sweeteners**—Nutra Sweet, Saccharin.
• **City, Well or Spring Water**

These are simply guidelines. If your particular system rejects this approach, it is your option to eat as you wish.
Except products containing white sugar; they must be avoided.

A Cassette tape is available which discusses the following subjects:
• **An expanded explanation of the diet itself, including recommended books and meal planning ideas**
• **What to expect as "normal" reactions when you are changing your diet**
• **And discussing the CanCell healing process**
This tape is available through **Nutrition Hotline** and costs $10.00 including shipping and handling. Send check or money order to **Nutrition Hotline, Post Office Box 2245, Farmington Hills, MI 48333-2455.**

* * *

The new holistic approach strongly recommended by Sopcak is part of his new departure from the old Entelev. His advocacy of strict diet restrictions, along with forbidding tobacco, is not deemed important by Sheridan and constitutes an important part of their disagreement about what makes their hypothesis work.

Mel Kramer, in Dayton, Ohio, has been tracking about 100 cancer patients who have used or are using CanCell. His assessment, based on conversations with CanCell patients over the past nine years, supports Sopcak's holistic theories. He indicates that 90 percent of the patients he talks with are doing well, but that their success depends upon a positive attitude coupled with strict diet, a no-smoking atmosphere and careful observation of some rules about electricity. He has learned that people who use electric blankets or water beds with electric heaters develop illnesses that an M.D. cannot diagnose. When they are eliminated, people get well. He warns about the effects of electrical vibrational frequencies from television sets, electric clocks at a bedside, computer monitors and high-tension electric power lines near homes. Ours is a world filled with electrical appliances and they are emitting damaging frequencies. When Kramer questions patients about such appliances in their environment, and they follow his advice to eliminate or protect themselves from them, he notes that they get well. He believes we need more physicists in medicine and fewer chemists.

Patients were required to use a Reorder Form when requesting a new supply of CanCell. It consisted of one page, printed on both sides, that included a short personal assessment of their progress. See Document No. 12, page 125.

Sopcak personally stopped taking orders for CanCell when the volunteers took over that duty. All new requests for CanCell were then made verbally to the:

CanCell Request Line 1-313-684-5529

Contacting the CanCell Request Line was always very difficult because there was a steady stream of calls being made and a busy signal was the usual response. People report having to redial (an automatic redial phone is suggested) continuously for several days before getting through.

ATTENTION! Do not reorder until you have been on this bottle for EIGHT weeks. We need complete, detailed input on your progress. Thank You.

CanCell Reorder Form

To Reorder CanCell, you must provide us the updated information. This form is only for people who are currently in our files. If it's been more than two years since you've used CanCell, you will have to initiate a new request verbally to Mr. Ed Sopcak
(313) 673-3643 between 11 am and 3 pm eastern time, Monday through Friday.

Name: _____ Date: _____

Street Address: _____

City, State, Zip: _____

Age: _____ Phone: _____

Type of Cancer or Condition Requesting CanCell For:
_____

Date First Diagnosed: _____

Previous Treatments: Chemotherapy   Diet & Supplements
(Circle those that apply) Hormone Therapy   Radiation
                          Other _____

Name and Address of Medical Doctor who Diagnosed your Condition:
_____

Name & Address of current doctor:
_____

Date Began CanCell: _____ Date Began This Bottle: _____

Since you began CanCell, or since your last bottle, what have you noticed? Ex: Pain, appetite, weight, energy, sleeping habits, skin color, circulation, waste material, or any other changes.
_____
_____
_____

What changes have been noted through medical exams, scans, blood tests, x-rays?: _____
_____
_____
_____

It would help tremendously if you could provide us with any medical documentation that you can.

How well have you been following dietary guidelines?
     poor ☐   fair ☐   good ☐   excellent ☐

How have you been following your time schedule for the CanCell itself?
     poor ☐   fair ☐   good ☐   excellent ☐

How have you been taking your bromelain glutathione, and/or BHT?
     poor ☐   fair ☐   good ☐   excellent ☐

In general, how have you been following the entire suggested program?
     poor ☐   fair ☐   good ☐   excellent ☐

Other Comments: _____
_____

7
Conclusion

Medical Service Industry results vs. CanCell results. A time for judgment. A fair, impartial testing is needed.

What drives cancer patients to use CanCell despite the fact that the American Cancer Society "strongly urges individuals with cancer not to seek treatment with this product"; the National Cancer Institute refuses to test it using a protocol of specific time guidelines essential to its success, thereby insuring its failure; the Food and Drug Administration will not approve it because of the NCI faulty reports and a U.S. federal court issued an injunction to stop its manufacture and distribution? The answer is that several thousand people, by word of mouth, have circulated the news that CanCell works, without side effects.

Critics argue that dying people will grasp for anything that promises hope and, of course, that is true. But upon close examination, CanCell does not appear to follow the usual methods of advertising and delivery that most unorthodox treatments have offered over the years. The circumstances surrounding CanCell, from its basic hypothesis to its unique free distribution, are so different from the usual offerings that it deserves investigation.

Innumerable unorthodox cancer treatments have been touted over the years. They all have had this one characteristic in common: like traditional treatments, they are expensive. They almost always involve clinics and physicians who demand premium prices for their services, just as traditional treatments involve expensive hospitals and physicians.

CanCell, and Entelev before it, has always been provided

free of charge. There never has been a charge for the material or its delivery and there is no expensive clinic or hospital stay required for its use. Neither Sheridan nor Sopcak ever have realized any financial gain for their efforts and both proclaim they never will accept any. That fact alone makes it unique.

Most unorthodox treatments, sooner or later, have been abandoned by their followers. They have failed because they have not produced the results patients seek, a cure for their cancer. Traditional treatment has also failed to cure cancer; but it is sanctioned by the ACS and the NCI, so the medical service insurance companies pay the bill for it. Patients accept the protocol because of the insurance money, although they survive their miserable last days coping with debilitating side effects. They don't know what else to do.

Sopcak claims to have several thousand testimonials from patients who credit CanCell with saving their lives without side effects. This simple demonstration of patient satisfaction should be enough to influence the medical community to take a very close look at this formula.

The American Cancer Society has been supporting cancer research for eighty years, since 1913, and has spent 1.4 billion dollars in the process. Their total budget for 1990-91 was $367,793,000 and only 26.2 percent of that, or $96,362,000, went for research, in spite of the fact that research was the prime reason for establishing the ACS. Most of the research money went to the same old people in charge of the same old research institutions that are tracking the same old treatments that haven't worked in the past and show no evidence of working in the future. Doesn't it seem reasonable to assume that the ACS can spare a few million dollars from their budget of $367,793,000 to test a cure that has been testified to by thousands of patients over the past fifty years?

After examining the no-cure record of established researchers, isn't it reasonable to conclude that something is seriously wrong with either the methods being used, the premise upon which the research is based, or both? Isn't it about time to listen to some other voices?

Sheridan and Sopcak challenge the accepted definition of what cancer is. If the establishment is wrong about this basic concept, a cure will never be found through establishment research. If Sopcak is proved right in his belief that cancer and all collagen diseases are caused by chemical or electrical vibrational frequencies and can be cured by changing those frequencies, we will enter a whole new era of medical treatment. It will be an era based upon the findings of Albert Abrams, M.D., whose 1920s findings were really the beginning of the system of Radionic Diagnosis which followed. Isn't this worthy of investigation?

We need to establish a National Cancer Registry where patients report the real outcome of their cancer treatments. Patients, or their surviving closest relative, should be required to file brief accounts. Included should be the location of the cancer in the body, the kind of treatment used (surgery, chemotherapy, radiation, other) the date the treatment began and ended, and the number of months the patient survived after treatment began and ended. These simple facts could tell a great deal about the real success or failure of current treatments.

It is obvious that cancer research is very expensive and so is testing. Both are controlled by the ACS and NCI, who have more than enough money, and their choices are dictated by the medical service industry. The politics involved is unconscionable. There must be a grassroots effort made to influence these two agencies to finance the testing of CanCell.

How can this be done? You can write eleven letters to places of influence. Call your local library for specific names and addresses of your state governor, senators, and representative. Then sit down and write a simple, one-page letter and get it in the mail this week. Don't let the week pass without completing this small task. Then get ten neighbors or friends to do the same, asking each one they contact to enlist ten more people. Make your letter simple and to the point. Just ask that CanCell be given a fair and impartial testing. Mail a letter to each of the following:

The President of the United States, 1600 Pennsylvania Avenue, Washington, D.C. 20500

The Governor of your state (name and address from library)

Your State Senator (name and address from library)

Your State Representative (name and address from library)

Your U.S. Senators (names from library), Capital Office, U.S. Senate, Washington, D.C. 20510

Your U.S. Representative (name from library), Capital Office, U.S. House of Representatives, Washington, D.C. 20515

The President of the American Medical Association, 515 N. State Street, Chicago, Illinois 60610

The American Cancer Society, 1599 Clifton Road N.E., Atlanta, Georgia 30329-4251

The National Cancer Institute, 9000 Rockville Pike, Bethesda, Maryland 20892

The Food and Drug Administration, 5600 Fishers Lane, Rockville, Maryland 20857

Then write a letter to Mr. Sopcak letting him know what you have done. All this can be done for less than $5 and a few hours of time.

Mr. Ed Sopcak, P.O. Box 496, Howell, MI 48844

Two very important issues are at stake in the CanCell

controversy. First, patients are being denied their freedom to choose the kind of treatment they want since the federal court injunction. Second, the world is being denied the possibility of a sure cancer cure because there has been no valid testing. This is because the mediocre leadership controlling medical research in the U.S. refuses to alter or suspend their outdated rules in the face of disaster. They are part of the problem the whole world wants solved. They simply do not understand cancer or the cancer patient.

We must accept the fact there is much about this world that we do not fully understand but which is just as real as if we did. We must begin to apply that philosophy to deal with cancer. We must begin a controlled study of volunteer cancer patients who will agree to use CanCell instead of traditional treatment and see what happens. It is as simple as that. For those who say we would be assigning those patients to quackery that would result in their death, I say let the patients look at the record of traditional treatment and choose for themselves.

It is appropriate to remind the powers that control cancer research in the U.S. of the famous quotation of Judge Learned Hand:

> "I beseech ye in the bowels of Christ, think that ye may be mistaken." I should like to have that written over the portals of every church, every school, and every courthouse, and may I say of every legislative body in the United States. I should like to have every court begin, "I beseech ye in the bowels of Christ, think that we may be mistaken."

Perhaps that should be written over the portals of every medical research center, medical school and the offices of the American Medical Association.

Epilogue

Interviews with CanCell users. CanCell and the U.S. Court

While writing this book, I talked with dozens of people from all over the country. These were cancer patients; physicians, dentists, and nurses; hospital, clinic, and medical school personnel; HIV and AIDS activists; medical researchers; medical laboratory technicians and family members and friends of cancer victims. All had unique stories to tell. Many patients told their stories in voices filled with the emotion that comes to people who have experienced being near death. I spoke with caregivers who had supervised the dying of a family member or friend and with professionals who treated patients in hospitals. I listened as an indignant "quack buster" spewed invectives condemning all alternative medical treatments, including CanCell. A medical school professor told me he knows CanCell works, but he doesn't want to get involved.

I was assisted in my undertaking by John Van Denover of Cedar Rapids, Iowa. He became interested in CanCell after reading a letter to the editor in the Cedar Rapids *Gazette* written by a CanCell user who had been denied further use of the material she believed saved her life due to the FDA-instigated federal court ruling of November 19, 1992, forbidding Sopcak to manufacture or distribute it. Van Denover was intrigued by the possibility of there being an existing cancer cure and angered that patients were being denied their freedom of choice in seeking treatment. He decided to do something about it. He began by calling the letter writer and then Sopcak, who told him about this book I was writing. His cancer education got into full swing as he contacted elected and appointed officials who referred him to established cancer organizations. Then he took off on his own, recording information from referrals he gathered with each encounter. He became a CanCell activist demanding, from anyone who would listen, that a clinical testing of the material be accomplished as soon as possible. He recorded phone interviews with a number of cancer patients and sent them along to me.

Of course, the medical service industry looks with disdain on patient testimonials, referred to in scientific circles as "anecdotal" accounts, worthy of little or no credibility unless backed by established methods of testing and record-keeping, complete with explanations of how and why the treatment worked. Cancer patients, on the other hand, listen attentively to stories of people who are living despite having been told by their physicians that they were doomed to die within a few months. Patients facing death are more concerned about the success of the treatment than the how and why of the success.

All of the physicians with whom I spoke admitted that their patients were, indeed, free from cancer after having used CanCell. All of them also asked that I not identify them by name, and all of them said that they would not recommend CanCell to any other cancer patients. In all fairness, we should be reminded that physicians who use any methods that are contrary to accepted medical practice run the risk of being sued for malpractice because the basis for malpractice is the use of methods that are not the accepted standard practice by the majority of physicians at the time and place of the use. Even though there has never been a case reported of any injury, death or adverse side effects from the use of CanCell, all of the physicians with whom I spoke were careful to tell me that they did not want to be identified and they simply could not recommend the use of CanCell. Most fear being ostracized by their peers and hounded by state and federal authorities.

Most patients stated that when their physicians found them free of cancer after using CanCell, those doctors reasoned that they had been misdiagnosed in the beginning and they really never had cancer. That was despite the fact that they had all the symptoms of cancer, as diagnosed by accepted traditional scientific examination, including tissue biopsies, and they had been given the traditional cancer treatments including surgery, chemotherapy or radiation. All the patients laughed in disbelief at the misdiagnosis explanation offered by their physicians.

Most of the patients interviewed spoke about their lost faith in the medical establishment. Many are convinced that there is a conspiracy to withhold CanCell from the public in order to protect the multi-billion-dollar cancer industry. Without exception, all had trusted and believed in the infallibility of their physicians prior to their use of CanCell. All were in the care of duly licensed M.D.s and had specialized diagnosis and treatment by licensed oncologists. All, even though they were lying at death's door and had been told they were terminal, were skeptical when they first heard of CanCell. They reasoned that if it were a valid treatment all physicians would surely know about it and would see to it that it was used on them. They turned off their traditional treatment and turned to CanCell only when they became convinced that they were going to die anyway. Since it was free, they had nothing to lose.

Many of the patients interviewed expressed a strong belief that a divine providence had interceded for them, sparing their life by presenting them with CanCell. In fact, they often said they were alive because of the grace of God, Ed Sopcak, and CanCell, in that order. Such references to divine intervention by devoutly sincere patients led some of the professionals from various cancer industry institutions to make sarcastic, disparaging remarks about religious fanatics when discussing CanCell patients, much as Jim Sheridan had been ridiculed when he claimed his invention of Entelev was divinely inspired.

The speed of recovery varied considerably among the patients, but all realized they were feeling better within two weeks after starting to use CanCell and were cancer-free within two to four months. Some were seriously damaged by the chemotherapy or radiation treatment they received prior to using CanCell, however, and surviving relatives told stories of how two of these patients died cancer-free, eventually succumbing to the side effects of the traditional treatment they had received. The relatives were convinced that if these patients had been given CanCell before the traditional radiation or chemotherapy they would have survived.

They talked of the side effects of chemotherapy that included hair loss, painful sores in the mouth and on lips, body sores, loss of appetite, weight loss, extreme fatigue, nausea, kidney or liver failure, and depression. Radiation added partial paralysis to one patient.

For those interested in personality profiles, I would report that every patient with whom I talked exhibited a spirit of hope, an independent sense of courage and belief in their own convictions, a natural curiosity and intelligence that drove them to investigate their illnesses, a sense of humor, and faith in a divine providence. All were thankful to be alive and were filled with a kind of missionary zeal to spread the word about CanCell. Some expressed the belief that surviving cancer taught them the true meaning of life and the experience was the best thing that ever happened to them. These cancer survivors are a special kind of people.

Contrary to the demand to remain anonymous by the physicians interviewed, patients were so anxious to tell their stories of triumph that it was hard to get them off the telephone! They supplied names of other CanCell patients, who in turn gave us more names and the lists grew and grew. They all readily agreed to having their names used, anxious to spread the word and save more lives. Included here is a brief listing of some of the people with whom we talked. Behind each name is a familiar story of the pain, fear, and expense known to every cancer patient, but with an unfamiliar ending of survival and a return to quality life due to their CanCell treatment. These patients have no official documentation and no evidence of double-blind studies or any other accepted standard medical proof of the efficacy of their CanCell treatment. They don't know why CanCell worked for them. All they know is that they are alive.

Charles Gilbert, Sr., of Sylba, North Carolina, was diagnosed with prostate cancer that had spread to the bone. He was told there was nothing that could be done to help him. He started taking CanCell and felt relief within one week. After six weeks his physician could find no evidence of cancer. He continues with six-month checkups and remains free of any clinical signs of cancer. He reported that his doctor "was interested in CanCell at first. Then when I told him he could get it for other patients, he said, 'No.'"

Robert Young of Dexter, Missouri, was diagnosed with lymphoma of the bone marrow and leukemia. He was treated with chemotherapy, developed pneumonia, and almost died. He suffered nerve damage in his feet and legs, causing constant severe pain. A second series of chemotherapy treatments again resulted in pneumonia. He decided to take CanCell in 1989, and after two weeks his symptoms, including the severe pain, were gone. Now he has blood tests every three months and remains cancer-free. He gave his physician literature about CanCell but never got a response from him. Now he worries that the court ban depriving him of continued use of CanCell will cost him his life.

Ed Bertsch of Sturgis, Michigan, had surgery to remove his appendix and part of his colon, diagnosed as cancerous. Another surgery to remove fifteen lymph nodes was performed, and he was warned that the cancer would return within two years. A third surgery was performed to relieve adhesions causing severe constant pain and colon blockage. He decided to take CanCell and within ninety days the pain was gone and there was no trace of cancer. He said he receives many phone calls from people who have heard about his recovery, "pleading" for information about getting CanCell.

Jean McElwee of Lakeland, Michigan, was diagnosed with ovarian cancer in February 1988. She had a hysterectomy but was told the tumor involved ruptured before the surgery, causing "floating" cancer cells that required chemotherapy. She was so debilitated by this treatment, which included using chemicals to combat nausea and left her body tissue feeling like a sponge and her veins collapsed, that she decided to stop the treatment and go home and die in dignity. A friend persuaded her to try CanCell and she started using it in July 1988. Seven weeks later she went for a blood test and her cancer count was down from 86 to 6. After three months there was no sign of cancer and she had no side effects. Soon she will have been cancer-free for five years, and she believes, "If it wasn't for Mr. Sopcak I wouldn't be here."

Virgil J. Boss of Jenison, Michigan, told the story of his involvement with CanCell used to treat his Hodgkin's disease. His oncologist advised him that the disease was in stage three when discovered and involved lymph nodes from his neck to his groin. He was advised that a six-to-eight-month regime of chemotherapy would give him a 60-percent chance of survival and that there was no other medical treatment available. He took the chemo treatment for about two and a half months, until he read that chemotherapy causes cancer. He confronted his oncologist with three questions: Does chemotherapy cause cancer? Where can I expect it to start in me? How soon can I expect it to start? His oncologist replied that he didn't know the answers to those questions. When Mr. Boss told him that he intended to start using CanCell, the doctor took a bottle of CanCell out of his desk drawer and said, "You mean this stuff?" He then said that he had eight or ten patients who were either using or had used it. Boss said his oncologist "never really bad rapped it," and agreed to follow his progress, which he has done ever since Boss started using the CanCell on August 15, 1988. He took it for one and a half years, then stopped after being tested "clean." Boss says, "I'm doing great, continually testing clean." He adds that he has become very interested in the study of cancer treatment and has spoken with many patients in the U.S. and Canada over the past four and a half years. He said that the majority of his contacts who have taken CanCell are alive and doing well or are cured completely. By contrast, of those who trusted their physicians and followed conventional treatment, only one or two percent are alive. He told about how he tried to pay Sopcak for the CanCell but was turned down, a familiar story. He concluded, "I'm a firm believer in CanCell. I wish I knew how to make it, 'cause I'd give it away."

Alice Lahrke of Colon, Michigan, was diagnosed with lymphoma on her liver, lungs, and pancreas, found on a body scan in July 1986. She had been in extreme pain and unable to walk since May of that year. She had seven partial chemotherapy treatments, causing hair loss and blisters in her mouth and on her lips. She heard about CanCell in October 1986 and started using it on October 10. She said that when she told her physician that she was going to take CanCell, "he got mad at me and said, 'You'll be back in three months in worse shape than you were when I first saw you.'" After using CanCell for ten days, her appetite came back, the pain steadily lessened, and she started walking again in February 1987. She has continued using CanCell ever since and never went back to any doctor until she was hospitalized with acute bronchitis in December 1991. At that time the physician who originally treated her asked if she was still on CanCell and, when she replied that she was, he said nothing. She said she has now lost faith in doctors and believes, "CanCell saved my life. Chemo and medications were killing me." She worries about not being able to get more CanCell when her present supply runs out.

Bob Sakal of Dayton, Ohio, was diagnosed with stage-four melanoma and given two years to live. He had tumors on his left knee and back removed. He heard about CanCell and told his oncologist, who was the head of the Cancer

Society in the area, about it. He said, "He wasn't very interested." Mr. Sakal started taking CanCell in July 1991 and continues to do so. He has "no sign of cancer now" and his "health is very good." About Sopcak, he said he would accept no payment for the CanCell and "I admire the man tremendously. Everyone who has had a life-threatening situation wants to help other people and I would like to help him."

Roma Fowler of Newcastle, Pennsylvania, was diagnosed with a melanoma on a toe. A team of oncologists pondered about whether to remove the toe, part of the foot, or the foot above the ankle. They told her that if they couldn't stop the growth she would have between four and six months to live. They told her that only surgical removal might cure her; chemotherapy or radiation would be useless. They removed the toe, and three weeks later the melanoma returned. One of the oncologists then recommended chemotherapy and she questioned this, reminding him of their earlier statement that it would not be effective. He denied their having said that. Shortly thereafter, in May 1990, she started using CanCell without supervision by a physician. The growth slowly diminished in size, leaving discolored scar tissue. In December 1990, she again visited an oncologist after being advised that a family history of colon cancer indicated that she needed a consultation and evaluation. This oncologist also examined her discolored foot, and she believes that he mistook the remaining scar tissue for returning melanoma. He warned her that nothing, including "Chemotherapy, radiation, or that chemical [CanCell] you're taking will do any good." He wanted to take off her foot. She refused and continued to use the CanCell as the blackened areas of scar tissue surrounding the melanoma site slowly continued to go away. A biopsy in January 1993 revealed no cancer. She believes, "Mr. Sopcak saved my life. . .I would have been dead a long time ago if I hadn't gotten the CanCell."

Philip Bates of Kinsman, Ohio, was diagnosed with

cancer of the bladder. He had surgery to remove the cancer, followed by chemotherapy, two times. Each time the cancer returned, and after the second surgery and chemo treatment his oncologist recommended that the bladder be removed. By this time he had heard about CanCell and decided to try it. After four months, there was no sign of cancer. That was three years ago. Mr. Bates is checked regularly at a V.A. hospital and remains clinically free of cancer. He said, "If it wasn't for him [Sopcak], I wouldn't be here today. . .I am totally sold. It is what they designed it to be."

Bill Browning of Sturgis, Michigan, was diagnosed with pancreatic cancer and given six months to live. He was told chemotherapy or cobalt might help, but he refused both. He started using CanCell a week later, on March 15, 1988, and continued with it until December 1991. Following Sopcak's suggestion, he quit smoking when he started using CanCell. He has a physician following his progress but is most impressed with the fact that "I'm still living." He is eager to recommend and defend CanCell and Ed Sopcak against attacks by the medical establishment who call alternative medical practices "quackery." He says, "I know better; I'm living proof."

Mrs. Jean Claar of Sherwood, Michigan, told about the cancer ordeal of her deceased husband, Veldon. He was diagnosed with stomach cancer on April 14, 1987. Nine days later he had surgery that removed his stomach and part of his esophagus, along with lymph glands. He was given two months to live. He started taking CanCell on May 29, 1987. In April 1988 he was suffering pain that he believed must be a re-occurrence of the cancer and went to the Mayo Clinic for consultation. There the cause of the pain was diagnosed as adhesions from the previous surgery, and he underwent another surgery to correct that condition on April 14. Later he received a letter from the surgeon telling him that there was no sign of cancer present during the surgery. Mr. Claar sent a copy of the Mayo

Clinic report to his local physician and that doctor sent a reply in which he stated, "I think it is miraculous that there is no evidence of re-occurring carcinoma, given the history. . .Maybe we should look more closely into CanCell." Upon hearing that he was free of cancer, Mr. Claar stopped taking CanCell on June 29, 1988, because he was told that he needed and was given intravenous mega-vitamin therapy to augment the poor nourishment he was getting as a result of the surgical removal of his stomach. This vitamin therapy, Mrs. Claar believes, "just fought against the CanCell," as Sopcak predicted it would and, three months after stopping the use of CanCell, Veldon Claar died. Mrs. Claar believes, "If he'd had the CanCell in the first place and not had the operation, he'd still be here." As it was, he lived one and a half years of good-quality life after being told he had two months to live. The cause of death was given as "starvation and fluid in the lungs."

And then there is Elonna McKibben of Warren, Ohio, diagnosed with Glioblastoma Multiforme, stage four, in October 1989. This is a rather rare (estimated about 200 reported cases per year) cancer that develops rapidly and takes the lives of 95 percent of its victims within two years of invasion. Usually it is found on the brain and affects the nervous system. Elonna was in the eighteenth week of a quintuplet pregnancy when she began experiencing extreme hip pain that resulted in severely limiting her physical activity. Two and a half weeks after delivering her five babies on September 9, 1989, four of whom survive in good health today, a CAT scan revealed the cancerous tumor on her spine. Doctors gave her six months to live. Two days later an MRI more clearly defined the earlier diagnosis, and she underwent surgery to remove the tumor on October 12. Four days later the neurosurgeon informed her that they couldn't get all of the tumor; it had runners that would send out more cancerous growth; and there were free-floating cells that would get into the spinal fluid and form new tumors in the spinal chord or brain. They recommended an experimental bone marrow chemotherapy that they predicted would destroy the immune system and would require her to live in isolation while this system regenerated. They could offer no guarantees but suggested that she undergo this treatment as a sacrifice to medical science in the hope of helping future victims. They also offered the option of radiation treatment that they predicted would eventually render her a paraplegic but would afford her from three to six months of extended life. When she received this prognosis, she was lying in bed after the surgery, with no feeling from the waist down, unable to even roll over without assistance. She couldn't keep food down and was developing other infections. She started making plans to undergo the radiation treatments, but changed her mind and decided to try CanCell, starting on November 12, 1989.

She immediately experienced the traditional results predicted by Sopcak, eliminating the egg white-like waste through frequent vomiting and diarrhea and an almost continual runny nose, along with profuse perspiration. At the start of the third week of CanCell treatment, she suffered a blood clot problem that threatened the loss of a leg and sent her to the hospital. She agreed to hospital treatment only if she could continue the CanCell treatment, which was increased to double doses, administered every three hours for five days. At the end of the week she was sitting up in bed, eating and experiencing reduced fever. She went home from the hospital after eight days, still unable to move herself in and out of bed, but still alive. In December she was able to go Christmas shopping in a wheelchair and soon started physical therapy that enabled her to stand alone. During the second week of January 1990 she started to learn to walk again. She had a CAT scan on February 5, scanning her lumbar spine, that revealed no more cancer and another on February 20, scanning the brain, cervical and thoracic spine with the same results—no sign of cancer. She decided that she didn't want to risk any more exposure to radiation and has declined further involvement with traditional medical testing or experimenting. She said, "I've been alive longer than anyone else ever lived with this type cancer. I don't need doctor's reports. I'm still alive. . .I basically reclaimed my life." She continued the CanCell through December 1991. She still has extensive nerve damage as a result of the surgery and walks with a cane, but has been taking care of herself and her family since March 1992. Her surgeon is now reported to have said that the fact that she survived indicates that the tumor was probably benign to begin with. He claims to have sent a prominent cancer expert pictures of the tumor and that expert declared it benign. Elonna wonders at this, believing that the biopsy should have settled that question immediately following the surgery. On September 13, 1991, he sent her a letter telling her that he had seen news reports of how well she and her babies were doing. He recommended that she return to standard care and have an MRI to evaluate her condition. This letter was followed by a phone call from his office offering to set up an appointment. She remembers that when she refused radiation treatment and told him she was going to use CanCell, he warned her that if she did something that he didn't prescribe he would not continue to treat her and as a result of that conversation she had no contact with him since November 1989. She continues to refuse traditional medical care. Her main concern now, after her desire to care for her husband and children, is to do what she can to promote freedom of choice in medical care for everyone. She said, "I would like for every citizen to have the right to choose."

Reflecting on the dozens of interviews, I was most impressed by the attitudes of physicians involved in cancer treatment. These people, by their selection and training, are obviously believed to be among our most intelligent citizens; and yet they appear to be a very intimidated class of individuals. Seemingly unable to evaluate treatment for themselves and accept reality as presented in their patients, they almost never recognize successful treatment that is not sanctioned by the medical service industry. They almost never admit to having made an honest mistake. Don't they know that we all make mistakes and the gravest mistake anyone can make is to deny an honest mistake? Many blame our malpractice laws and legal system but, in fact, our legal system provides for excusing honest mistakes. Is it the malpractice insurance industry? Would physicians be better off dropping the insurance, informing their patients that they have done so, promising to do their best and having them sign waivers? Shouldn't they finally admit that sometimes their failures are not due to what they don't know, but rather to what they do know that isn't so?

As of November 19, 1992, Edward J. Sopcak has been ordered by U.S. District Judge Bernard A. Friedman to stop making and distributing CanCell. (See Document No. 13, page 142.) This action came as a result of Sopcak's ignoring a similar decree issued on January 17, 1990. Sopcak believes both actions were taken illegally because neither was initiated by any wronged party. That is, nobody has ever accused him or CanCell of causing any injury whatsoever and he believes only a wronged party may instigate such legal action. However, although he ignored the earlier order and continued to manufacture and distribute CanCell free of charge, he declared that he "has been forced under threat, duress and coercion by Judge Bernard A. Friedman," to comply with the latest one and will pursue the matter via the courts through an appeal of the decision. Sopcak is a serious, brilliant student of constitutional law and is preparing and presenting his case as a private citizen. He is not using the services of an attorney, claiming that he can't find one who is familiar with or understands the constitutional law upon which he is basing his defense.

Representatives of the medical service industry continue their attempts to discredit CanCell by claiming that it has never been clinically tested using a double-blind study; therefore it has not been proven effective. They refuse to recognize patient testimonials, even though those testimonials are complete with medical records provided by licensed physicians and oncology specialists. The idea that patient testimonials are not scientific and therefore have no merit reflects the medical establishment's practice of not listening to patients when they do not present themselves according to traditional establishment theory. Physicians simply will not believe their own eyes. In fact, the methods that the medical service industry representatives often declare "scientific" are faulty in themselves. James Carter, M.D., writes in his book *Racketeering in Medicine* on page 6:

> The double-blind study was developed to prevent bias in agricultural research up in Canada. To test the effects of fertilizer on crop yields, Canadian agriculturists planted two patches. The experiment was "double-blind" because neither the harvester who measured the crop nor the researchers knew which patch was fertilized and which one was not, eliminating the element of subjective bias. Double-blind studies were never meant to be used as the sole criterion for determining scientific truth, however.

The double-blind study has no place in the testing of CanCell. Since it has never been used to test any other cancer cure, why has it been cited as the only acceptable test for CanCell? A double-blind study that would treat half of the patients with CanCell while furnishing the other half with a placebo would place the placebo half of the patients in a position where they would go untreated, assigning them to certain death, rendering such an experiment unconscionable.

CanCell should be clinically tested in the traditional manner, using volunteers. We need to call for cancer patient volunteers who will choose to use the establishment's dictum of surgery, chemotherapy, or radiation in as many different cancer locations in the body as we can find patients to present them. We need to call for volunteers to use CanCell in the same type of patients. By doing this we test both the traditional methods and CanCell. Then we follow the progress of these patients through the rest of their lives, checking and comparing the results. It is as simple as that; and it is as scientific as the art of practicing medicine will ever get.

Historians have recorded that Benjamin Rush, M.D., one of the signers of the Declaration of Independence, had argued that the Constitution should make a special provision for medical freedom as well as religious freedom. He believed that, if it were not included, the time would come when medicine would organize into an undercover dictatorship. As we all know, such a provision for medical freedom of choice was not included in our Constitution as a basic right, and we are now suffering the predicted consequences. Not only are our citizens being denied access to the medical treatment of their choice, they are being denied information about what is available. Our medical service industry, once the respected world leader in research and development, is being controlled to the point where its leadership has abdicated its sacred trust. Independent medical research has moved to more fertile grounds, outside the U.S. Can we get it back? Of course we can; but not without dramatic political changes that will come about only when our citizens demand them.

UNITED STATES DISTRICT COURT
EASTERN DISTRICT OF MICHIGAN
SOUTHERN DIVISION

UNITED STATES OF AMERICA,

      Plaintiff,

vs.

EDWARD J. SOPCAK,

      Defendant,

_____/

CIVIL NO. 89-CV-70559-DT

HONORABLE BERNARD A. FRIEDMAN

JUDGMENT AND ORDER OF CIVIL CONTEMPT AND FOR ENFORCEMENT OF PERMANENT INJUNCTION AGAINST EDWARD J. SOPCAK

Plaintiff, United States of America, having filed a petition for an order to show cause why defendant Edward J. Sopcak, and his agents and representatives Diane Petosky, d/b/a Nutrition Hotline, and Bonnie Sue Miller, d/b/a Solution for Health, Inc., should not be adjudged in civil contempt of the Decree of Permanent Injunction ("the Decree") entered by this Court on January 17, 1990; and a memorandum of law and declarations in support thereof; and the parties having appeared at a hearing on November 13, 1992, and the Court having considered the petition and the supporting documents and the evidentiary record in the case, and it appearing that the defendant Sopcak is violating and, unless found in contempt by Order of this Court, will continue to violate the Decree entered by this Court on January 17, 1990;

IT IS HEREBY ORDERED, ADJUDGED, AND DECREED that:

1.   This Court has jurisdiction over the subject matter and

over the defendant and his agents and representatives.

2.   The Order to Show Cause states a cause of action against the defendant and his agents and representatives pursuant to 18 U.S.C. § 401(3).

3.   Defendants Bonnie Sue Miller and·Diane Petoskey are not adjudged to be in civil contempt of the Decree issued by this Court. The defendant, Edward J. Sopcak, is adjudged to be in civil contempt of the Decree issued by this Court.

4.·   Defendant Sopcak shall come into full compliance with the Decree immediately. To effectuate such compliance, the defendant, within fourteen days of the date of this Order, shall undertake the following measures, among others that may be deemed necessary and appropriate:

A.   Defendant Sopcak shall provide notice to all of his donees, by first class, that he will no longer distribute articles of unapproved new drugs, that articles of unapproved new drugs distributed since January 17, 1990 violated a Decree of Permanent Injunction entered by this Court on January 17, 1990, and that such articles of drug will not be available in the future. A copy of such notice shall be provided to the FDA Detroit District Office, 1560 East Jefferson Avenue, Detroit, Michigan within five days of the time such notices are placed in the mail to consumers.

B.   Defendant Sopcak shall place a recorded message on his answering machine stating that he has been enjoined from distributing Cancell or any other unapproved new drug product whose distribution is enjoined by the Decree of Permanent Injunction.

   C. Defendant Sopcak shall report in writing to FDA's Detroit District Office by November 27, 1992 the actions he has taken to comply with the terms of this Order.

   5. The issue of costs shall be held in abeyance. Should defendant Sopcak violate this order, government counsel may seek attorneys' fees plus all other costs of this action, including investigatory and administrative costs, incurred in the investigation and prosecution of this case.

   6. This Court retains jurisdiction to enforce the provisions of this Order and the Decree entered on January 17, 1990, and for the purpose of granting such additional relief as may be necessary or appropriate.

   7. Defendant Sopcak shall appear before this Court personally on January 26, 1993 at 2:00 p.m. in Room 228 of the United States Courthouse to report on his compliance with the terms of this Order and the Decree.

   Defendant Sopcak reserves all constitutional rights, if any, under Section 1-207-8 of the Uniform Commercial Code.

Dated this _19th_ day of _November_, 1992.

                  BERNARD A. FRIEDMAN
                  United States District Judge

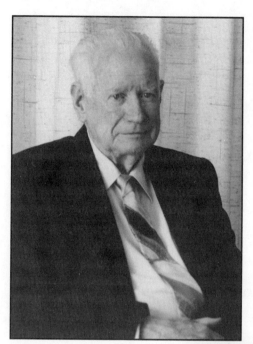

Jim Sheridan

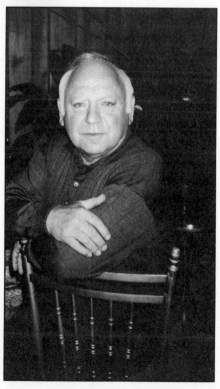

Ed Sopcak

About the Author

Louise Trull is a former high school English teacher who resides in Rockton, Illinois. She earned a B.S. in Education from Eastern Illinois University in Charleston, Illinois, and attended graduate school at Northwestern University in Evanston, Illinois. Her contributions to current issues and community welfare include a term on the Winnebago County Board of Supervisors in Illinois. Her own experience with cancer led her to research the topic extensively, culminating in this, her first published book. She has three grown children and is currently pursuing a law degree at The John Marshall Law School in Chicago.

Mel Kramer
PO Box 5982
Dayton, Ohio 45415
Ph 937-277-6076

Hampton Roads publishes a variety of books on metaphysical,
spiritual, health-related, and general interest subjects.
Would you like to be notified as we publish new books in your area of
interest? If you would like a copy of our latest catalog, just call
toll-free, (800) 766-8009, or send your name and address to:

Hampton Roads Publishing Company, Inc.
891 Norfolk Square
Norfolk, VA 23502